To Our Readers:

INTRODUCING

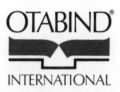

OTABIND®

INTERNATIONAL

"The Book That Lies Flat"
— *User Friendly Binding* —

This title has been bound using state-of-the-art **OtaBind®** technology.

- The spine is 3-5 times stronger than conventional perfect binding
- The book lies open flat, regardless of the page being read
- The spine floats freely and remains crease-free even with repeated use

We are pleased to be able to bring this new technology to our customers.

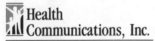

Health Communications, Inc.

3201 S.W. 15th Street
Deerfield Beach, FL 33442-8190
(305) 360-0909

OTABIND®

INTERNATIONAL

The Netherlands

STAYING SANE

When You Care
For Someone With
Chronic Illness

Melvin Pohl, M.D.
and
Deniston J. Kay, Ph.D.

Health Communications, Inc.
Deerfield Beach, Florida

Library of Congress Cataloging-in-Publication Data
Pohl, Mel.
    Staying sane: when you care for someone with chronic illness:
a guide for caregivers/by Melvin Pohl and Deniston J. Kay.
    p.   cm.
    Includes bibliographical references.
    ISBN 1-55874-251-4
    1. Chronically ill — Care — Psychological aspects. 2. Cargivers
— Mental health. 3. Stress management. I. Kay, Deniston.
II. Title.
RC108.P64   1993
649.8 — dc20   92-40511
                                                   CIP

© 1993 Mel Pohl and Deniston J. Kay
ISBN 1-55874-251-4

Publisher: Health Communications, Inc.
              3201 S.W. 15th Street
              Deerfield Beach, Florida 33442-8190

Cover design by Andrea Perrine
Illustration by Bonnie Rheault

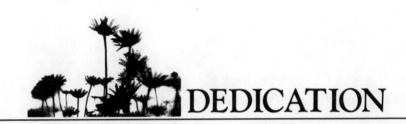

DEDICATION

We dedicate this book to
all caregivers.

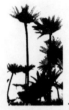ACKNOWLEDGMENTS

We acknowledge with gratitude the following people for their support and contributions to the manuscript:

All the people who were interviewed to create the vignettes, Ellen Ratner, Doug Toft, Mairz Davis, Annetta Brown and Gina Gross.

Greg Shea for the photographs.

And to Eleanor and Phil Pohl, Irene and Joseph Kay — for all they have taught us about caring.

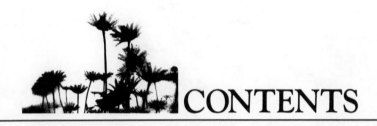

CONTENTS

Introduction ix

1. **BECOMING AWARE:** Monitor Your Insides 1

2. **ACCEPTING:** Meet Life On Life's Terms 19

3. **CONNECTING:** Make Contact With
   Other People And Yourself 33

4. **RELATING:** Gain Intimacy And Balance
   In Relationships 63

5. **JOURNALING:** Discover What You
   Already Know 79

6. **SELF-CARING:** Remember Yourself 97

7. **CHANGING:** Adapt And Heal 111

8. **CHOOSING:** Remember That You Are
   Not A Victim 129

9. **SUMMING UP:** Make Your "Master Map"
   For Caregiving 147

Endnotes 163

Resources 167

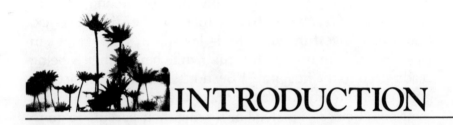

INTRODUCTION

IDENTIFYING WITH THE CAREGIVER

This book is for all the people who care for people with chronic illness (PWCI). It tells stories about caregivers of people with cancer, AIDS, muscular dystrophy and Alzheimer's disease. The principles and exercises in this book will also apply to caregivers of people with any chronic health condition such as emphysema, heart disease, chemical dependency, diabetes and mental illness, to name only a few.

We've written this book as a comprehensive guide for caregivers. It spans all phases of chronic illness (CI). These include the first frightening uncertainties of diagnosis, the caregiver's response to loss of health, vigor and independence of the person with chronic illness and the changes in self-image and self-esteem that all caregivers experience.

One key issue for caregivers is how to provide care and love without losing themselves in the process. The phenomenon of making another's needs more important than one's own has been referred to as co-dependent behavior: when caring becomes a necessity, an obsession or the desire to help becomes the need to control another person.

It is common for caregivers to feel so committed to helping that they lose sight of other things that are important to them. They feel responsible for others and they feel guilty if something goes wrong. Isn't this the ultimate in goodness and giving? Isn't it better to give than to take? If Dan is sick, how can I have fun while he is laid up in bed? How can Jackie be such an ungrateful child while her mother is being readmitted to the hospital? Why don't Paul and Rose act like good children? Shouldn't they take their ailing parents into their own homes — instead of forcing their parents to go to a nursing home?

Questions like these plague all caregivers sooner or later in some way or another. Some people believe that to be a good caregiver and a decent human being you must sacrifice everything. But what about the needs of the caregiver? What happens to feelings of anger and resentment?

This book helps caregivers find a balance along the spectrum of caring without being consumed. If they continue to give all the time, what will be left? We will introduce the concept of interdependence — the skill of loving and caring without being consumed. We will help you take care of yourself as a caregiver so you can take better care of the PWCI. We will provide techniques to enhance your sense of self while remaining aware of your own needs so that you don't get "used up" in the demanding role of caregiver.

Some caregivers call that "used up" feeling burnout. Burnout is a blanket term, useful for what it says and even more for what it leaves unsaid. Burnout is not just one feeling. Rather, it is a combination of feelings:

- Stressed much of the time
- Worthless
- Tired and out of energy
- Out of shape

- Emotionally out of control
- Constantly in the grip of negative thoughts
- Out of time
- Out of money
- Alone and disconnected
- Depressed
- Anxious about the future
- Used up.

We will provide strategies for getting past such feelings and for safeguarding your own health and well-being. We believe one of the keys to staying sane when caring for a PWCI is holding on to a healthy attitude and image about the illness. If you regard cancer, Alzheimer's or AIDS as a death sentence, then you commit yourself to sit in the very vestibule of death — listening for the death rattle, waiting for the end. If you do this, you miss the best part: the process of living in the precious time available, whether days, months or years.

If, however, you embrace life and look at the illness as a life challenge rather than a death sentence, the experience of caregiving becomes enriching, life-enhancing and productive. It is by embracing life that PWCIs actually live longer. This depends to a great extent on their willingness to fight, to live and to bask in the experience of living. What becomes important is the quality of life, each day taking on a meaning and significance that surpasses the realities of illness. PWCIs survive by committing themselves to finishing unfinished business. They truly find meaning by living with chronic illness.

For everyone, caregivers and noncaregivers alike, life's meaning comes in part from the very act of caring. As philosopher Milton Mayeroff notes, "In the sense in which a man can ever be said to be at home in the world, he is at home not through dominating, or explaining or appreciating, but through caring and being cared for." This book, this journey, is about living with another's chronic illness — and about living to the fullest.

THIS APPLIES TO YOU

We've written this book with a wide audience in mind. Caregivers are wives, husbands, children, nurses, counselors, physicians, parents, grandparents, friends, lovers, co-workers, volunteers. Often personal caregivers are professional caregivers as well.

More specifically, those who can benefit from this book include:

- People who care for someone who has a chronic illness. The list of diseases is long and includes Alzheimer's disease, cancer, heart disease, diabetes, AIDS, chemical dependency, emphysema, tuberculosis, hepatitis, herpes, arthritis, lupus, multiple sclerosis, neurological diseases such as muscular dystrophy and a multitude of emotional illnesses such as depression, anxiety and thought disorders.
- Professional caregivers including counselors, physicians, social workers, nurses, office personnel — anyone whose work deals directly or indirectly with PWCIs.
- Any person with a chronic illness — you may learn about your illness and about the people who care for you.
- Volunteers who participate in support groups and support organizations dealing with chronic illness.

CHRONIC ILLNESSES: COMMON GROUND

We mention a diversity of chronic illnesses because we want to invite you in, no matter what chronic illness has entered your life. This may seem a little abstract at first: If you're caring for someone with diabetes, for example, you might wonder how reading about people with cancer or heart disease could help you. This is a natural question. It's human nature to look for differences rather than similarities, to feel unique rather than connected. The key to this process is exploring your uniqueness while finding common ground with other caregivers. (We will talk more about the value of connecting and techniques for doing so in Chapter 3.)

This common ground comes from the very meaning of the words chronic illness. What is chronic? The dictionary defines it as "marked by long duration or frequent recurrence, always present, constantly troubling."

In short, to say that something is chronic is to say it may always be present. It never goes away. The opposite of chronic is acute, which means self-limited, or temporary. Illness or disease, in turn, is a process that alters the body's structure or function. Dis-ease means, literally, "not at ease."

Illness can be either acute or chronic. Colds, for example, are acute. They end and that's it — they're gone. Other infections are like that, too — appendicitis, hepatitis, pneumonia. Sometimes acute illnesses, such as hepatitis, can become chronic. That happens if the person who gets acutely ill (the host) is unable to fight off the attacking germ or condition. Even a cut or bruise can turn into a chronic condition, especially if it becomes infected. What's more, chronic illnesses can affect almost any system of the human body: connective tissue, the endocrine system, the immune system and many more.

Many of these chronic illnesses have common characteristics. They tend to involve alternating periods of wellness and sickness. The latter we refer to as relapses or recurrences. Most chronic illness is progressive — that is, over the long term PWCIs gradually get sicker. This progression may be totally unpredictable, sometimes slow and sometimes rapid.

Many people live for 20 years or more with these illnesses. And because the course and outcome of chronic illness are unpredictable people with chronic illness often feel powerless, "at the mercy of the illness" or as if they are "living on a roller coaster." At the same time, they can forget the other person who's along for the ride — the caregiver.

Most of the chronic illnesses we will talk about are *treatable* yet incurable. Many have fatal outcomes in some people. Many people with chronic illness are stigmatized. They feel shameful about their illness and so do their caregivers.

Many treatments for chronic illnesses can have serious side effects. With many chronic illnesses caregivers must make decisions about which treatment to take, leaving behind other options and facing the consequences of these choices.

All chronic illness affects the lives of the people with these illnesses — and those who care for these people. Often, depending on the relationship between caregiver and patient, the illness has an impact on emotions, finances, spirituality, social interactions and sex. When chronic illness is introduced into a family, for example, everything in that family may change and may never return to normal. Daily routines, future plans, friendships — all can be altered.

During our travels we've met and talked with caregivers across the country. We were struck by the universality of the plight of caregivers and the usefulness of certain ideas. We were equally impressed with the resilience of the human spirit when coping with the inevitable sequence of psychological adjustments to chronic illness: initially denial and shock, followed by depression and even despair, and gradually adjustment and acceptance. These stages are detailed in Chapter 1 and in our book *The Caregivers Journey: When You Love Someone With AIDS.*

Today there's growing recognition of the caregiver's vital role. It is seen in the hospice movement and in the rise in home health-care services, which depend on professional and lay caregivers. This makes sense. After all, caregiving in the home is more cost-effective than in a nursing home, hospital or hospice care. There is a new breed of caregivers, sometimes the elderly and ill themselves. And all of them need emotional support along the way.

The skills useful in living with CI are for everyone. We all have a terminal condition called "life." Chronic illness just brings universal life issues into clearer focus. This can be a gift if you can only learn to claim it.

As caregivers you will benefit by developing and using certain skills. Some of you may find yourselves using these skills naturally. You may have grown up in an environment where these skills were taught and affirmed, or you may have learned them as adults. For others the ideas may feel as foreign as wearing your left shoe on your right foot — awkward, uncomfortable, even painful. If these skills are, or become, a part of your nature, it will be more likely that you will call upon them throughout your journey.

The key skills illustrated in this book will be the corner-stones for the applications. Each chapter title names an action. We encourage you to take action as you read this book. Participate. Exert energy. We will suggest ways to respond to chronic illness that can help you manage your feelings and help you stop feeling like a victim.

Reclaim some personal power on the emotional roller coaster ride we call chronic illness. Even on a roller coaster you can learn different ways to decrease discomfort. You can close your eyes. You can ride with another person and talk about how you're feeling. You can scream. By all means hold on tight — or do you want to try riding with "no hands"?

The actions we recommend for caregivers include:

Becoming Aware

Naming and knowing what you are feeling, needing and wanting are critical tasks for a healthy caregiver. In order to become aware, you need to begin to monitor your insides and do a "needs assessment."

Accepting

Chronic illness presents caregivers with plenty of situations they don't like. Often it feels as if your internal gears are out of sync — grinding and scraping. It's painful. And sometimes the harder you try to make them work right and the more you force those gears to shift, the worse it seems to get.

Accepting is an art. It enables you to give up judgments. With chronic illness you come face-to-face with suffering, limitation, even death. It's easy to get caught up in fear, shock, anger and sadness. These negative feelings maintain the dissonance, the discomfort. When you stop trying so hard, the gears mesh more smoothly. Things are less strained. When you're willing to meet life on life's terms, you can discover a source of comfort that does not depend on health, income or other external conditions. This calls for getting help, slowing down, oiling the gears or even stopping the motor for a while to let it cool down and rest.

Connecting

This is making contact with others. We will focus on techniques of expressing yourself, negotiating, talking and, when necessary, fighting (fairly, of course). We will stress the importance of openness and honesty. Some caregivers find that the quality of the connections they make during the caregiving process is the essence of loving care.

Relating

When caring for someone with chronic illness, it is important to balance closeness to the PWCI with setting personal limits on one's involvement with the PWCI. We will assist caregivers in maintaining healthy distance and a sense of self in the midst of chronic illness. We will discuss the art of providing care without being consumed by the caregiving process.

Journaling

It is common for events and reactions to those events to become jumbled in people's minds. Often, people crowd a multitude of experiences into their days with a multitude of feelings in tow. Too often they emerge from the passing years with no clarity, central passion or source of direction. They feel lost; their experiences seem meaningless. If you feel this way, writing, journaling, organizing and developing ideas on paper may help you find your way. Writing can be more powerful than thinking and talking. By recording things on paper you make a commitment. It's also harder to be dishonest on paper since when you reread it, you have to see it again. Forgiving and letting go by writing it out can also be very healing.

Self-Caring

As a caregiver, you're entitled to care for yourself. You can do things that help you feel good. Avoid unhealthy behaviors. Take time out from your role as caregiver. All these options are good for you. In fact, they're essential. They will help you be an effective caregiver.

To safeguard their own well-being, caregivers need to exercise defense mechanisms in healthy ways. It is neither necessary nor possible to always be in touch with the intense emotions that accompany caring for one who is ill. Part of healthy denial is being able to identify "danger signals" that indicate a need for self-care. We identify *positive* denial and offer practical techniques to lessen our own suffering.

Changing

We will talk a great deal about changes that occur with the onset of illness. Many caregivers are tempted to keep things as they have been. They hold on. But, especially with chronic illness, the tighter you hold the more painful life becomes, and the more powerless you feel because things have already changed. In order to survive you must adapt and change with life as it happens.

As part of changing it helps to enlarge your repertoire of behaviors, activities and interests to avoid putting all your eggs in one basket. Businesses diversify in order to become

more financially healthy. Caregivers can apply the same principle to their emotional lives. In this chapter we explore
ways to go beyond perceived limits.

Choosing

Chronic illness introduces new variables. You will be faced
with countless decision points. You must choose or choices
will be made for you. Many of these choices are difficult.
The options and possibilities may seem inadequate — or too
plentiful. This chapter describes choicemaking and explores
ways to find health-promoting choices — choices that will
leave you feeling good about yourself.

Living with chronic illness is a process. That process takes
time — and in the end it is the process that is the most
important part of caregiving. You must make time in your
life and be patient as your experience as caregiver evolves.
We will look at ways people are caring, sad, angry, afraid.
We will look at what it means to want to give up — and
what happens next. We will also suggest ways to relax, talk
to others and anticipate changes.

HOW TO USE THIS BOOK

Don't feel obligated to "get it all" the first time through.
In fact, feel perfectly free to come back to this book from
time to time and take in only as much as you want. The text
is structured so that you can read it straight through — or
dip in anywhere you choose.

Please don't make this book another burden in your already burdened life. In fact, if you can gain more competence
with just two of the skills we mentioned — becoming aware
and accepting — you'll find yourself well on the way to sane
caregiving. Our suggestion is that you use *Staying Sane* as
one port in the storm of chronic illness. The reflection it
prompts can become part of your daily routine, much like
eating and sleeping.

This book is loaded with ideas and possibilities for action. Choose the ones that seem appropriate for you and your lifestyle. Everything you read here is a suggestion — nothing more.

You'll also find "applications" throughout — opportunities for you to follow up on the things about which you're reading. These are labeled "learning," "working with feelings" or "taking action." It's not required that you complete any of these exercises or journal entries. You may think of applications that never occurred to us — ideas that are far more powerful and appropriate for your situation. That's great. Our hope is only that using this book will make your life a little easier and make caregiving a lighter, more rewarding experience for you. If and when hard times come, we hope this book will help you through. When you apply ideas, when they come off the page and start working in your life, we hope you find life going a little better.

When do you start with your first application? Some people function better starting immediately. Others need some time to get used to the idea of change and may respond well to setting a deadline. Still others miss many deadlines and end up never changing.

We think a reasonable strategy is to start small. Take little steps at first. When overwhelmed by massive changes, taking a small step may be just enough. It is important not to be hard on yourself if you are unable to accomplish some of the changes we suggest. Try to be satisfied with little changes that gradually lead to new behaviors.

1 BECOMING AWARE:

Monitor Your Insides

In this book you will meet several caregivers and their PWCIs. The characters are composites of many caregiving families: Rose is the caregiver of her elderly parents, Michael and Elsie (who has progressive Alzheimer's disease). Mark is a caregiver for his lover Dan (who has AIDS). Stella and her cousin Lola are the caregivers for Stella's daughters Christine (stricken with muscular dystrophy) and Irene (who has diabetes), as well as her husband Ted (an alcoholic). Pearl is a caregiver for her daughter Rita (with Hodgkin's disease), Rita's daughter Jackie, who helps as a caregiver, and Rita's younger child Joey. Each of these characters will illustrate both different issues faced by caregivers and different styles of coping.

ROSE, ELSIE AND MICHAEL

Elsie and Michael were facing their future through a bead curtain of question marks. Elsie, aged 70, was stricken with arthritis and suffering from Alzheimer's disease. Her condition was deteriorating. Michael, a 76-year-old devoted husband, was being advised to put his wife in a nursing home. His doctor, son and daughter had been urging this for the past two years. Now Michael was becoming short of breath and having dizzy spells.

"What if you get another spell and are too sick to get up to feed Mama? Or what if she walks out of the condo and out of the building?" his daughter Rose asked. Rose, aged 50 and in good health, lived in New York City with her husband John and their son Brandon. Rose certainly did not want to burden herself by becoming the primary caregiver for her mother and father, but as a guilt-ridden daughter she was willing to spend part of the winter and some holidays with her parents. The years of pleading with her parents to relocate from Miami to New York City so she could be nearer to them had ended. Now there were strong urgings, verging on threats, to place her mother and, perhaps, her father into a nice nursing home in New York City.

"Brandon and I will visit you each week. And you can see your granddaughter Lisa and your great grandson. They'll come in from Syracuse. Syracuse is so close to the city."

But nothing worked. "I don't want to be with those old people," shouted Michael. "I want to walk on the beach each day with Mama. She loves the ocean. That's why we moved here. This is our home."

Rose called her brother Paul in Los Angeles and her parents' family doctor in Miami. The opinion was unanimous. Their father, Michael, was intractable. He would remain his wife's caregiver until one of them dropped dead. "It's impossible," lamented Paul, a book publisher in California. "How about trying a day nurse again?"

"The home health-care people refuse to send anyone over, Paul. The private nursing agencies refuse to send anyone again — ever. They've had eight private nurses walk out. They've been through seven cleaning women in three months. The people come and go. Ma and Pa are impossible. He's stubborn. You remember what happened to the last batch of help? They were lazy or dirty or drunk. They didn't speak English. They didn't understand directions. They were lousy cooks or they were thieves or they were too rough with Ma or they were not strong enough. And they were all argumentative and unreasonable — all 15 of them, Paul! Ma and Pa could have Betty Crocker and Hazel the Housekeeper and they wouldn't be satisfied."

"Look, we're intelligent people. There must be a way to convince them to give up the apartment and go into a nursing home. Unless they live with us — you six months and me six months. We both have room, you especially."

"Oh Paul, what a lousy idea. Pa and John fight like cats and dogs when they're together. Their personalities explode like firecrackers. I don't want my home turned into a war zone. Having them move in with us is out of the question," Rose sighed.

"You have much more freedom than I do, Rose. Why don't you spend more time in Miami with them?"

"You don't do anything in New York anyway," was the unspoken message! Paul felt he was being kind. He thought his sister was a very selfish woman.

PEARL, RITA AND JACKIE

Pearl was gathering some essentials into her daughter Rita's overnight bag, crying and wondering if she should call her grandchildrens' schools. Their mother was being taken to the hospital again. "I have to pull myself together," she thought. She blew her nose, a signal for all tears to return to their homes and families. Rita was coming out of the bathroom. "You'll need a dressing gown or two," Pearl said from the depths of the large walk-in closet, shaking her head while she bypassed several choices. "For God's sake, Mama, I'm going to the hospital, not to an April-in-Paris ball. Anything will do!" Rita replied.

Rita had been through so much the past few years. Chemotherapy had caused her to lose all her hair. Pearl bought her colorful head scarves and penciled in her daughter's eyebrows, and baldness would give way to wispy peach fuzz and eventually to the cropped look favored by Gertrude Stein and channel swimmers. But then there would be more chemo and more hair loss. Rita could endure the nausea which was almost unbearable, but always vain, she found the hair loss embarrassing and demoralizing. She refused to leave the house for a month. "I hate looking like a concentration camp survivor. I can't take the stares."

Pearl saw her role in all of this as rallier of Rita's sagging spirits, hence the scarves, the eyebrows and eventually, after much coaxing, a trip to the local mall.

Rita had been diagnosed with Hodgkin's disease when she was 30 years old. She had first undergone radiation treatments and surgery. The disease had remitted, but the stress of cancer put such a strain on her marriage that her husband of eight years left her and their two children Jackie, age 15, and Joey, age 10. Since getting sick again five years ago, Pearl and Rita's daughter, Jackie, have been her primary caregivers. Pearl had moved from New York City to her daughter's home in Los Angeles in order to give her hands-on care.

Pearl and Jackie have seen Rita through numerous stays in the hospital and her regular trips to the clinic for radiation. They've seen her through abandonment and divorce, depression and a dwindling social life. She had to relinquish her executive position at the television studio because of her illness — too many unproductive or missed work days. In the past two years, after a recurrence of the tumor, the doctors started chemotherapy, and Pearl and Jackie saw her through the treatments and the side effects.

Through it all Pearl turned everything to favor and prettiness. She talked in honeyed tones and always outwardly held out hope. She never ever showed frustration or impatience towards her daughter.

Jackie, on the other hand, was resentful and impatient. At times she was even petulant. She could not bring her friends around because Rita was sick so much of the time. All of her schoolmates were planning their sweet sixteen parties. Pearl advised Jackie that this was not the proper time to plan a big party. "Even though your mama will get better, it's best if we wait. There will be plenty of time for parties."

Jackie sobbed and through her tears shouted, "Sometimes I wish she'd just die!"

Pearl raised her fist with the impulse to strike the crying girl, restrained herself and shouted, "If I ever hear you say such a thing again, you can just get out of this house and never come back! Now go to your room! You make me sick!"

As Jackie ran through the house, Pearl broke into tears herself, amazed that she had come so close to hitting her granddaughter, something she had never done.

DAN AND MARK

Mark stared out the window. The yard was a gallery of bronzes, goldenrods and jades. Indian summer was hamming it up. Part of him missed New England, especially this time of year when the trees became showpieces. Within two hours Mark would be on a plane heading back to Phoenix, to his ailing lover, Dan, and to the drudgery and burden associated with caregiving. The couple had undergone many changes since Dan's diagnosis with AIDS six years earlier. For one thing, because of the chronic fatigue associated with his low T-cell count Dan was forced to quit his job, virtually reducing the couple's income by half. This required a major lifestyle adjustment. They had to sell their home situated in the desert on an acre of geographic elegance and move into a two-bedroom townhouse. This change was very painful, but it made sense. The couple had been unable to make monthly payments on their large home or to maintain the house and grounds.

Another change in the couple's lives was the all too frequent visits from Phyllis, Dan's mother, who now knew she had to announce her visits. When she first learned of Dan's illness three years ago, she'd fly in at whim for visits — storming in like Napoleon at Elba.

"Well, what fresh hell is this?" questioned Mark.

"It's Rosalind Russell playing Bella Abzug," chuckled Dan, still able to maintain a sense of humor.

"I'm here to see that as far as my son's care is concerned, things are running right," Phyllis barked, when confronted by the surprised and exasperated men.

Mark seldom needed her for caregiving purposes or for any other reason. When he needed "mental health" days or occasional long weekends, he'd call on Brenda, their neighbor. Brenda, understimulated, overweight, 39 and unnoticed, was a nurse at St. Joe's Hospital. When the AIDS ward opened and Brenda volunteered for duty, a whole new world opened up for her. The gay men paid attention to her, took notice of her attributes and made no mention of her ample hips and multiple chins. Those who were able did her hair.

Though she mingled with most of the men, she instantly bonded with Dan and Mark. She liked them because they both had the gift of gab and a gutsy sense of humor full of lift, wit, anecdote and personality. During the long periods of reconstruction after pneumonia, convalescing in the hospital and at home, Brenda would be there.

"I'd think you'd have enough of 'nightingaling' at St. Joe's — yet you come here to look after Dan," Mark commented appreciatively.

Brenda laughed, adding, "I'm also here to look after you, Mark. I'm worried about you. You should get away more often."

And Mark eventually would, even though he felt conflict about leaving Dan for days. "How can I think about having a good time when my lover is so sick?" he'd think to himself. At other times, Mark, feeling suffocated and over-burdened, would feel absolutely entitled to these get-away extended weekends. "After all, I'm HIV positive, too, and I have a low T-cell count. I have to make the most of my life. Our social life together has been limited for the past year. I'm tired of waiting on him like a servant. I'm tired of bickering. I'm still young and healthy and I want to go out dancing. I still have a libido. Dan doesn't want to dance; he doesn't want to have sex. Why should I deprive myself?" he tried to convince himself.

Sometimes Mark would be downright selfish in his deal-ings with Dan. He felt entitled when he'd walk into a room and switch TV channels from some educational news pro-gram favored by Dan to an inane sitcom featuring out-spoken teenagers with braces on their brains engaging in pitter-patter.

So life for Mark consisted of continuously balancing car-ing for Dan and making sure his own needs were met. Could the couple maintain and sustain the love and harmony they had had in their relationship all these years? Or would resentment caused by overwork, guilt and tedium prevail?

STELLA, LOLA AND CHRISTINE

Stella was eating a box of cheese crackers and looking at the piles of dirty clothes harboring wildlife. She glanced at her stupefied husband, Ted, drunk in his chair in front of the TV. He looked consumptively thin. His cheeks bore the hollows of ten years of TV dinners and suppers improvised from tins. She looked painfully at her daughter Christine, suffering with muscular dystrophy and recently confined to a wheelchair, and she looked at Irene, her three-year-old diabetic baby, sleeping in the crib in the kitchen. Christine was so lonely and depressed. The one playmate who was kind enough to visit and spend time, who was not put-off by Christine's paralysis, had moved with her parents to another part of town.

Stella was lonely, too. Ted offered little or no emotional support. He escaped his problems through TV and beer. Stella prayed that he'd stop drinking — just as she had. She'd been a drug user for years, but got clean through treatment and counseling. She remained clean and sober through Narcotics Anonymous (NA).

Until last year, when 13-year-old Christine became wheelchair bound, Stella would attend NA three times a week and would often speak at local conferences — telling her story about drug addiction, her history of picking lemons in the garden of love and her search for sobriety. Now Christine could no longer look after the baby when Stella went out. In fact, someone had to look after Christine. Like Christine's, Stella's own mobility was now limited, but in a different way. Having Christine available as a built-in baby-sitter had afforded Stella a few hours of independence each week — time for NA meetings and coffee with her sponsor. Christine, though young, had also been able to help out with laundry and house cleaning. Now the burden of all the household chores fell on Stella. Her burden was compounded by Christine's neediness.

Besides a weekly NA meeting, now the only diversions and bright spots in Stella's and Christine's lives were the frequent visits from Stella's cousin, Lola, who was also in recovery. Lola had a history of co-dependent behavior. Stella knew this. That's why the laundry remained undone and the beds unmade. She knew Lola would pitch in immediately and help her with the housework. She'd also cook a hot meal for Christine and Stella, and for Ted, too — if he was around.

Lola tried to bring some joy into the family's dismal life. "You have to have hope, Stella. Do something for yourself," Lola would advise. "You have to find your own sunshine," she'd say.

But was there any hope for Stella? The family's destiny looked dark and tragic.

These vignettes illustrate several different types of problems facing caregivers of people with chronic illnesses. Rose, with both parents ailing and stubborn, feels a myriad of emotions, the most important of which are guilt, guilt and guilt. Lola embraces the whole family as her project and rises to the occasion. Pearl is ever present, ever watchful of her daughter's needs and has forgotten her two grandchildren in the process. And Mark has his hands full juggling his own needs with those of Dan, his ailing lover. The first step for each of them is to slow down or stop, listen to their insides, and develop an awareness of how they are feeling, what they are thinking and what needs to be done.

STARTING NOW

To start feeling the healing effects of awareness, you can start today — right now — by working with two things: paying attention and naming.

Paying attention means noticing what's going on in your life — in your relationships with others and inside yourself. Try to train yourself to be more precise and less judgmental. As a caregiver, you may tend to focus on the needs of the PWCI. It's important to monitor and respond to your own needs as well. As you do, your skill at becoming aware will increase dramatically. This book offers many opportunities to develop that kind of awareness.

Naming is the other important function in developing awareness. In the name lies power. Giving something a name — whether an illness or an emotion — is one means of accepting it, and will later enable you to do something about it.

STAGES IN LIVING WITH CHRONIC ILLNESS: A ROAD MAP FOR AWARENESS

The following stages are artificial. They may or may not apply to the caregiver and may or may not always apply to certain illnesses. These stages are helpful to caregivers as organizing principles, milestones on the journey, examples of what others experience. Many caregivers find reassurance and a sense of balance knowing that they are not alone in the process. Identifying stages helps make sense of the experience and helps reduce feelings of powerlessness!

Action nouns reinforce the fluidity of each stage. Each stage occurs over time; it evolves. Transitions between stages may happen gradually and gently or abruptly and painfully.

Stage One: Discovering

The first stage for caregivers is discovering. This is the time you first learn of an illness in a loved one or in someone for whom you care. It is the time of diagnosis — the first glimpse of what's to come. You project the future, often based on your limited knowledge and experience with chronic illness. For example, before learning that her mother had cancer, Jackie only knew about the disease from her friend's grandmother who died three years earlier. So when Jackie first heard the word cancer, she immediately equated it with death.

During this stage, most people's first response is shock. They shut down. They run from the facts. As the shock subsides, they are left with emotions like anger, fear, shame, hopelessness, sadness and despair.

It is during this stage that many people do what they know best: deny the feelings, bottle them up, walk away or hide. Why? So they can carry on, continue to function. This may be perfectly logical for some people, who learned to deny feelings while they were growing up. They think that if they don't feel the emotional intensity of their feelings, they are able to function better, at least in the short run.

The discovering stage explores those early feelings and the ways you may have learned to cope with them. Some of you may find you got stuck there. At the time, you had to deny and block out the way you felt. In order to get unstuck, you need help.

The other major issue in Stage One is disclosure — who to tell, whose news this is. Jackie's mother has the diagnosis of cancer — Jackie wants to talk about it. Her mother, Rita, doesn't want her to tell! What a dilemma! This book explores these issues and some of the difficulties caregivers face in this stage. Then it presents exercises to help clarify the issues, facilitate communication and enable compromises to be reached.

Stage Two: Adapting

After discovering comes adapting. After the PWCI and the caregivers pass through denial and ride the emotional roller coaster associated with the diagnosis, they must then adjust to the illness. So as a caregiver you change and adapt.

If, as a caregiver, you successfully adapt, you will survive. If you merely resent and resist the changes, you are apt to suffer and experience much more pain. This stage requires the most work from you.

Stage Three: Coasting

After you adapt, you enter a new and almost unexplainable state of calm. It's called *coasting*. It's like the eye of the hurricane — the winds are blowing all around you. But at least for a time you feel safe. You have adapted and have established a new equilibrium, a new norm, a new routine. Life with illness has become regular.

What are some of the different things in your new routine? Perhaps daily vomiting or diarrhea, cough and other symptoms of the PWCI. Michael has to change Elsie's wet bed linens each night; Mark has to feed Dan when he first comes home from the hospital. You may have to bear reduced income, mood changes, daily injections, medications, visits to the doctor or clinic. Your new life with chronic illness now includes all these things and they become part of the routine.

More than any other stage in your journey, the theme of this stage is adjustment to loss. It's an awkward paradox, chronic illness and regularity. Shock and tragedy have entered your life; you feel new limitations and get used to them.

And life is regular. Chronic illness has become part of your life. Sickness has become typical, expected. It feels a little like balancing while standing in a moving subway car — distributing your weight and shifting constantly, you've become accustomed to the underlying clackity-clack of the wheels on the tracks. Many people stand and read the paper during such a ride. Others may have to work harder to keep their balance. People react differently. How you react depends upon who you are.

Stage Four: Colliding

If there's a sudden stop, sharp turn or collision, then the equilibrium is disturbed. Many become off-balance and may fall. This is Stage Four or *colliding*. In Stage Four, it is common to re-experience Stage One emotions all over again. It's back to square one, only you have to adjust to a new set of realities.

Probably the most difficult factor in chronic illness is the unpredictability of what's to come. "How long?" is the common question caregivers ask the physician. The honest answer with most chronic illness — with AIDS, with Alzheimer's, with cancer — is "We don't know. Probably a long time, but maybe not!"

What's going to happen? Is Dan going to waste away? Is Stella going to be able to get pregnant again and have babies or is the risk too great? Will Elsie get worse and not recognize her family? Will Rita come home from the hospital — this time?

In the next section there will be some exercises on handling unpredictability and making contingency plans. By planning for some terrible outcomes, you may find that your fear will be diminished.

Application 1: Learning

This exercise provides one way for you to define what the abstract term — chronic illness — means in your own life.

First, name the chronic illness in your life.

Next, write down everything you know about it. If this sounds overwhelming, then just make an outline of the major topics. Such topics might include physical symptoms, required medication, emotional effects, traditional treatments, nontraditional treatments and so on.

Read over what you've just written and look for any gaps in your knowledge. Write two or three questions that describe what you'd like to know.

PEARL, RITA AND JACKIE

When Pearl and Jackie tried this application, they discovered far more than they anticipated.

Pearl was called in to talk with the social worker from Jackie's school. Jackie had been cutting classes. If and when she attended school, she acted out — disregarding teachers' requests, arguing with classmates or, at times, withdrawing. Her grades were slipping.

Pearl told the social worker about the situation at home: Rita's Hodgkin's disease, frequent trips and prolonged stays in the hospital, the aborted sweet sixteen party, evenings and weekends left at home to baby-sit while Pearl coped with hospital tedium and maintained the vigil.

Pearl, uncoaxed, acknowledged that her granddaughter's and grandson's needs had been put on the back burner for longer than she wished to admit. Her daughter's care and comfort came first.

The social worker made some suggestions, and Pearl, jolt-ed by her granddaughter's truancy and failing grades, re-solved to at least try to implement some of them.

That afternoon Pearl broke her pattern and rearranged her schedule. She surprised Jackie and Jackie's brother, Joey, with an announcement that she was not going back to the hospital that evening. The three of them would have dinner together at 6:30 P.M. rather than 5:00 P.M., as they had been doing for the past six weeks since Rita had been readmitted to the hospital. Although Pearl fretted about leaving Rita alone that evening, she knew she had to reset her priorities, at least for that night. The food felt like ashes on Pearl's tongue.

After dinner Pearl told Jackie about the call from the school social worker and started to cry. She admitted how neglectful she had been of her grandchildren's emotional needs. Indeed, the children were always well-dressed, fed and neatly groomed, but TLC had certainly been in short supply from the old woman since her daughter had taken a turn for the worse.

The exercise suggested by Mrs. Goodwell, the social worker, called for Pearl and Jackie to sit down together, talk and write.

The words "Hodgkin's disease" were seldom, if ever, used in the household. "Mama's sick" or "Your mama's not well" were the only messages given to the children about their mother's frequent bouts with the illness. But this evening, at the suggestion of Mrs. Goodwell, the words had to be enunciated and written. Pearl and Jackie talked and wrote about it as suggested. Here is what they came up with:

1. Hodgkin's disease is very serious! Many people have died from it.
2. It is cancer of the lymph nodes.
3. It affects mostly young women although men get it, too.

4. There is no real cure, but it can be arrested for long periods of time (five years or more), which is considered a cure.
5. The primary treatments are chemo or radiation therapy which can cause the patient to get very sick.

Jackie, now interested, wanted to know what drugs were used to treat the disease. "Why do the drugs make Mama so sick?" Pearl said she once knew, but it was so technical she forgot. "But if it's important to you, baby, we'll try to find out together." Jackie also wanted to know how many people had died from Hodgkin's each year.

Jackie wrote out each of her questions as directed, neatly and carefully. She was surprised at how pleased she felt to be able to spend time with her grandma. She now knew how much she had been missing her grandma's love and nurturing.

Pearl said they'd need to get the answers to these and other questions — and they could add questions to the notebooks she had bought that day, recording all the new information they'd be gathering.

They decided that tomorrow they would ask one of the interns at the hospital about the drugs used for chemotherapy and their horrible side effects. She and Rita chuckled when they thought of those interns — they all tried to look so serious despite their comic youth. Pearl would write the answers down in her notebook. Jackie was to call the American Cancer Society when she got home from school Monday — yes, she promised Pearl she would return to regular school attendance — to request information and some pamphlets about the disease. The grandmother and granddaughter wrote their assignments down in their notebooks.

Application 2: Working With Feelings

Now label the illness, but not with its technical or medical name. Instead, write about the way it feels. This is an important step toward becoming aware of the illness — even making friends with it.

To complete this step, list three words that capture your feelings about the chronic illness. Or, if you like, just jot down some words or phrases from the list below. Feel free to add more words.

- Sad
- Angry
- Tired
- Okay part of the time
- Up and down
- Helpless
- Confused
- Irritable

- Limited
- Afraid
- Sensitive
- Vulnerable
- Open to others
- Closer to tears
- Closer to other people
- Closer to the person I care for

Pearl was very proud and sensible, and she rarely indulged in self-pity. But she felt sad that her daughter and grandchildren had to go through all of this. She told this to Jackie and urged Jackie to express her own feelings about Rita's disease. Jackie wrote in her notebook that Hodgkin's was (1) long, (2) never-ending, (3) the center of their lives, (4) draining for all of them, (5) filled with the nightmare of hospitals, doctors, clinics, tests, vomiting . . . and she resented all of this. So she felt scared, sad, tired and angry. She verbalized these to her grandmother and there was a long pause.

A realization hit Pearl and Jackie at almost the same time — like a thunderbolt. Rita's disease was consuming all of them, Pearl, Jackie and young Joey, not just Rita. And all of them had suspended living. No fun, no joy, no parties, no studying, no friends . . . just Hodgkin's disease. Pearl realized that she must not let Rita's illness hold her grandchildren back from life. It would take Pearl a while longer to realize that this reasoning also applied to her.

Application 3: Taking Action

List two or three actions you could take to answer the questions you listed in Application 1. Make these actions concrete — specific enough to write down in an appointment book. For example, you could call your physician. You could check the phone book for organizations that focus on the chronic illness you named. Perhaps there are organizations, such as Al-Anon, for the caregivers or relatives of people with this illness. If so, you could contact these organizations.

List your actions along with a time and date for doing them.

Application 4: Learning

Look for other materials on coping with life change, especially as they relate to loss or illness. Two particularly helpful books to begin with are *On Death and Dying* by Elisabeth Kubler-Ross and *Anatomy of an Illness* by Norman Cousins.

This chapter has presented some of the issues that caregivers experience, and has explored the importance of becoming aware of them. The journey toward becoming a healthier caregiver has begun. It is by developing awareness that caregivers are able to assess their situation, accept what is and make changes if they need to.

2 ACCEPTING:

Meeting Life
On Life's Terms

How can caregivers most readily make sense of their lives with PWCIs? Meaning can be found in the fullest experience of the moment. Picture yourself looking through the lens of a camera — capture the moment — live in the snapshot. Focus on what's really special about this moment, right now! And now. And now again. And again now. This is what living life in the present is about — being totally here, available for whatever comes up. Part of this process is letting go of remoteness, of dissatisfaction about what isn't, of absent-mindedness, of self-contemplation. All of these behaviors function to remove you from the moment.

Like looking through a camera at an instant in time, shoot the picture again and again, moment by moment. Each moment becomes unforgettable, joyous, rich, full of itself and, yes, painful, too.

The same process can work with pain. Lean into the pain
— move with it — be with it — experience it to its fullest.
Stephen Levine talks about "bestowing loving attention on
the pain, on the fear, on the anger." That doesn't mean to
ignore it, nor to meet it with hatred and resistance, but to
allow it to become a part of you in its fullest sense, with
kindness, and to let it go as it comes to you.

WHAT TO DO WHEN THE WORDS END

When a person is present to the process, one of the things
he or she may discover is that words are sometimes awkward or useless. Sometimes they're hard to express. Caregivers don't have an answer for this suffering and pain.
They can't cure illness and sometimes they're not sure they'll
survive the whole experience alone. Their loved ones are
here today — who knows what tomorrow may bring.

Words are only one way to communicate. Talking may
actually block comunication. If a caregiver is present to the
process, at times they can just stop talking and hurt. They
can find meaning in that experience by being present *in the
pain*. The pain is the reality at that time, and then it passes.
PWCIs are often deprived of touch — a potent and comforting force. Sometimes touching, holding a hand, is the most
meaningful form of communication.

You may get confused. When you admit your lack of
answers, you strip yourself of the facade of the supposed-
to-be-all-knowing caregiver. You become yourself. And in
that moment when you offer yourself as you really are, you
give people a chance to get to know you, to meet you where
you stand. That's when your friends, family and the PWCI
can truly connect with you.

Admitting confusion, touching, being silent, smiling, crying, just being — these are tools that can serve patients as
well as caregivers. You can speak to others not only through

what you say and do, but through who you are, by touching, by listening, by merely being present.

LET GO OF "WHY?"

One of the first questions caregivers are tempted to ask is "Why?" Why chronic illness? Why now? Why her? Why me? Loved ones struggle for answers to these questions and assume that the PWCI wants such answers also.

They also want to know how and who. How can I make sense of what is happening to me, to us? How can I live with this? How will I get through this? Who will be with me as I do?

"Perhaps we don't really need answers to 'Why me?'" thinks Mark.

"We just need to know that it is so. And, somehow, that it will be okay, that we will survive, that I will survive." Sometimes a person just needs to sit still and hurt.

So much of caregiving, it seems, is about waiting. Waiting for treatments. Waiting for insurance matters to be settled. Waiting for medications to take effect. Waiting in hospital rooms and doctor's offices. Waiting for a vacation, a chance to rest, a chance to sleep. If caregivers investigate their everyday experience, they may well find all the signs of prolonged waiting — sighing, tapping feet, humming, counting, impatience — are focused on their thoughts for the future.

Yet the waiting — and the willingness to do so — is a sign of caring. When you're willing to wait, you're really saying that you're ready to go through the experience of chronic illness with the person you care for. Waiting is another aspect of staying present to the process.

PHASES OF ACCEPTANCE

Acceptance is a concept that has been studied and written about for many years. Acceptance is a source of strength and power for caregivers who learn to harness its energy.

Accepting is an action that refers to enduring, approving or receiving with consent. In the case of caregiving, it means approaching chronic illness as a given — now what's to be done about it?

Chapter 1 suggested that people and their caregivers go through a series of stages in living with chronic illness. In many ways those stages describe what happens on the outside: the diagnosis of chronic illness; changes in relationships, jobs and living arrangements; seeking treatment; remissions and relapses in the illness.

People with chronic illness and their caregivers also take a series of steps "on the inside" toward accepting what's taking place "on the outside." These steps are called phases and are designated with letters — A, B, C and D. Many times these phases describe the way the caregiver thinks, feels and chooses to act in response to chronic illness.

The first phase is *learning*. Learning means gathering information that will help build a data base about the chronic illness you're dealing with. In Phase A you use your intellect. You reason, compare, judge and evaluate what chronic illness and caregiving are all about. That means reflecting on how you've coped with problems in the past and considering alternative solutions. Rita and Pearl made a start in Chapter 1.

Phase B is *working with feelings*. In Phase B you use your heart and your guts. This phase may evoke painful emotional responses that you need to experience. This book explores ways and introduces exercises to help you know the feelings, experience them, express them and let them go, if and when you're ready. It will be important to get help from others during this phase as Mark does from Brenda.

After learning and feeling, it is time for Phase C, *taking action*. You make choices, changes. When you take action, you change reality — you reclaim personal power for yourself. Taking action enables you to assert your will, your needs and your wants.

The final phase is one everyone should experience. It is called *accepting*, Phase D. This phase involves the ultimate form of human adaptation to "life on life's terms." Acceptance means a growing sense of serenity, an inner strength that steadies you even when events take a turn for the worse.

What allows this serenity to develop? First, as explained in Chapter 1, you must maintain your awareness. With a foundation of awareness, you can work your way toward acceptance: learning, feeling and taking action. These phases may help you turn something that seems unmanageable — caring for a PWCI — into something that's more manageable — living one day at a time with a loved one who is sick.

There are tools you can use to work through each phase of acceptance: forgiveness, prayer and meditation, letting go, relaxation, developing gratitude and more.

ACCEPTANCE AND CHANGE
WORK TOGETHER

Acceptance is not the same thing as giving up. Surrendering in this case does not mean throwing in the towel. Acceptance is an important step toward change. The irony is that once you've fully accepted your current condition, you've already taken a step beyond that condition.

Acceptance means letting go of the desire to change things that can't be changed. It means adapting to what is. It means changing from expectations — rigid scripts about how you want the future to turn out — into expectancies. Expectancies are preferences about how you want your life to develop. Preferences, however, are simply that. They do not describe what has to take place before you can be happy. Rather, they indicate how you'd like things to turn out.

For example, you'd like the person you care for to become stable in health, perhaps even cured of chronic illness. But even with this expectancy, you acknowledge that

this person's health may get worse. What's more, you resolve to find ways to feel secure and at peace — even if the
worst takes place. You find that happiness, instead of being
something that life brings to you, is an outlook that you
bring to life.

Accepting does not mean giving up, becoming passive or
feeling hopeless. Instead, accepting means seeing what is,
not what should be. It means standing back and seeing all
the anger, sadness, mistakes and grief clearly, without judgment. It means letting go of images about the long-suffering,
patient and perfect caregiver you "should" be. If you start to
base your life as a caregiver on these ideas, you will find a
little more acceptance coming into your life each day.

THE PATH TO ACCEPTANCE

The rest of this chapter consists of applications, ways to
apply what you've read so far — to learn, to work with
feelings and to take action. Choose one of the following
applications to complete within the next week. Then come
back and try some of the others. Write your responses in a
notebook, on cards or on scrap paper.

Application 5: Learning

Think of a time in your childhood when somebody who was
close to you was sick. What was your reaction? Were you al-
lowed to stay around or were you taken away? What kinds of
responses did people have? Write about them now. For example, Stella remembered, "When I was six years old, Dad disap-
peared from us for six weeks. When he came home, he was
different, weak, unsmiling. It wasn't till I was grown up — ten
years later — that I understood he had a heart condition caused
by high blood pressure and smoking too much. His drinking
hastened his death. I thought it was something I had done that
made him sick. I felt responsible and horribly guilty."

What was your experience of your own illness? Think back to
when you were sick for the first time you can remember. Did

you complain? Did you stay home from school? How were you taken care of when you were sick?

How was illness viewed in your family? Was it used or misused? Rose recalled, "I used to get ill instead of dealing with my feelings. Today illness can still be a weapon for me: If you aggravate me, I'll get sick or better yet have a heart attack. I use sickness as a weapon."

Application 6: Learning

Now think a little more about the role illness played in your family as a whole. Did people talk about it? How did they carry through with it — deny it, use it, make the best of it or exaggerate it?

Application 7: Learning

Now write about the role of illness in your present life. Do you approach illness in any of the same ways you did as a child? Or have you learned new ways of responding to illness?

Next, focus on the PWCI. Spend a few minutes "walking a mile" in that person's "shoes." Write a letter to one of that person's good friends describing what it's like to have a chronic illness. Be sure to write in the voice of the PWCI.

When you're done, consider reading what you've written to the PWCI and asking for that person's responses.

Your PWCI can also do something like this, writing from his or her perspective, as Dan does in the following example.

DAN AND MARK

When Dan and Mark felt certain emotions, they wrote down what they wanted. Some of Dan's entries looked like this:

This afternoon the pain in my leg was so great I felt afraid. I wanted assurances from Mark or my doctor that the pain would subside as it had in the past. I wanted pain pills from my doctor. I needed hugs from Brenda and Mark. I asked for all of these things and got what I needed.

Today I was pissed off because Mark was grumbling that he needed to share the secret with Tommy and Jay. I needed to know that Mark respected the fact that this was my illness and that I considered the matter personal and private. I was angry because Mark never seems to have enough support even though I know he has plenty. Why must the world know? I'm also afraid that Tommy and Jay will back away and drop us. They are such a fun couple to be around and when I'm feeling fine, we all have a great time together. I need Mark to promise to hang on a little while longer and not divulge my *secret.*

Application 8: Taking Action

This exercise demonstrates a standard approach to solving a relationship problem. You'll find many variations on it throughout this book, so it pays to learn the basic approach first.

1. Get out a pen and paper. Be prepared to spend at least 15 minutes writing. Have plenty of paper on hand and make yourself comfortable. Be in a place where you are not likely to be interrupted.
2. Jot down some notes about any relationship problem that is troubling you. Describe the situation as a newspaper reporter would, answering the questions Who? What? When? Where? How? Stick to the facts of the situation — the things that an outsider could see or hear. Be as objective as possible.
3. Describe your response to the situation. What do you know about it? What do you feel? What action, if any, have you taken or considered taking about this situation?
4. Now separate what's "you," what's "him or her" and what's "us" in this situation. If you're not sure, ask someone you trust for help.
5. Now visualize a solution. See the problem as already being solved. Describe what's changed in your relationship as a result. Picture yourself talking to the other person, and use all your senses. What do you see, hear, feel, touch? It's important to just let your mind work freely. Don't filter out any image that seems unlikely or impossible.
6. Write down the key points that arose in your visualization. Note these quickly without stopping to edit them. When

you're done, look over your list. Do any of the items point to actions you can take today? What are they? As for the other items on your list, what actions could you take to bring these solutions one step closer to reality?

7. Finally, choose one action you intend to carry out and write down when and where you will take this action.

Here is an example from a situation that responds to this exercise:

DAN AND MARK

Tommy and Jay, a gay couple whose company Dan and Mark enjoy, were extending a dinner invitation for the third time. And once again Dan and Mark had to decline because Dan was not feeling well. Tommy and Jay did not know about Dan and Mark's illness. "Do we dare disturb happy friendships with bad news?" Dan asked Mark. More to the point, Dan did not want tons of people to know he had AIDS and that Mark had tested positive for HIV. In conservative Arizona AIDS was rapidly turning into an inquisition, as rife with terror and scapegoats as any launched by Rome in the fifteenth century. Dan and Mark had experienced rejection by a few of their Boston friends. They had also seen friends with HIV positive status lose family, clients and jobs. Dan and Mark had oceans of unresolved rage reserved for people who ran from the sick, abandoning friendships, but they also saw that plague and panic were inseparable.

So for now Tommy and Jay's dinner would go unsampled by Dan and Mark. The men profusely thanked Tommy and Jay for the invitation as they white-lied about a previous engagement. A few minutes later, Brenda called from work to find out how her friends were feeling. She was working the 3:00 to 11:00 P.M. shift at the hospital.

"We're feeling lousy. It seems when he's sick, I'm sick or depressed, too. Dan has major diarrhea again and is weak and tired. We're also arguing again over whether to tell

Tommy and Jay. Dan is insistent on keeping his illness a
secret. We had to refuse still another one of their invitations.
And I really wanted to go, but we're staying home as usual.
Thanks for asking," Mark whined.

Mark, who'd been in a support group for partners of
people with AIDS, had picked up a few coping skills and
Brenda suggested he use some of them . . . quickly. She
hated to see him suffer and his whining depressed her. So
Mark hung up and began detailing in his journal:

Problem: Dan's pain is my pain. When he feels worse, so do I.

*Typical response: When asked how I'm feeling, I find myself saying:
"We're feeling lousy — Dan has diarrhea again and is weak and
tired. We'll be staying home again."*

*What's Dan? His pain — his feet hurt — his diarrhea — three
times so far today and it's not even 9:00 A.M. — can't get too far from
the john — his AIDS — low T-cell count — his sadness because he
has pain and is tired of sitting on the toilet — his uptightness and
shame about AIDS — his fear of rejection.*

*What's me? My headache — my impatience — when will he feel
better? My feelings of inadequacy and frustration — I can't do anything to make him better — my sadness because he's sick — my fatigue
because I didn't sleep well after he left the bedroom when he was sick
— my boredom — I'm feeling that life is passing me by, that I'm
giving up so much to sit home with him night after night. When will
he feel comfortable telling the guys? My sense of isolation — I want
to share my feelings with Tommy and Jay but he won't let me.*

*What's us? Neither of us knows how Dan will feel tomorrow. Both
of us feel powerless and scared sometimes. We're both isolated, frustrated, angry.*

*Solution: I could get a friend to stay with Dan on Friday nights so
I could go out with friends. I don't have to be gone a long time — just
a nice relaxed dinner will do. I see Dan and I talking about this. I'm
relaxed about it and so is he. He understands and says, "Go out and
enjoy yourself." I can smell the dinner — pizza, of course, at a local
joint that I love and he hates. Brenda's with Dan and they're okay.*

Actions I could take: Talk to Dan about this today. Tell him I want some time alone so I have more to bring to him when we're together. Call a friend and set a date to go out for dinner. Define a time when Dan agrees to let me tell Tommy and Jay. Until then, let it go, in fact, don't even discuss it. I just hope he doesn't say, "Two years."

Application 9: Working With Feelings

Define what you want when you feel a certain emotion. Doing so can help you ask for help instead of being stalled by negative feelings. For example:

When I feel . . .	I want . . .
angry	a listening ear, not to be angry
afraid	hugs, reassurance, space
sad	company, fun.

Consider asking the PWCI to do this exercise also.

Application 10: Taking Action

Look at the effects of the way you speak, the language you use in diagnosing and treating chronic illness: salvage, fatal, should, have to, can't, terminal, deadly.

For the next 24 hours notice the way you speak about chronic illness. Jot down the words and phrases you use without judging yourself.

Now see if you can think of more powerful and positive ways to speak about chronic illness — ways that open up more possibilities and choice. For example, say that you find the words "I have to" cropping up in your speech frequently. Can you use "I want to" in any of those situations instead? Other examples — instead of dying, look at living each moment.

Finally, choose one new positive word or phrase you plan to use in talking about chronic illness.

WORKING WITH ANGER:
MAD AND LOOKIN' FOR TROUBLE

Anger is one emotion that's often "up front" for caregivers. It deserves some special attention as you begin your path to acceptance.

Anger comes to the surface in a myriad of ways. Listen to them:

I just woke up mad today for no good reason. It's a grey day. I slept wrong. She snored all night. Hell — I'm just angry and I don't need a reason. It's my right!

My life sucks. It's way too hard and I don't deserve this.

So what if I snap at the kids or the dog? I've got feelings, too.

I'm sick. I can't face another day. We had a good time last night, but this morning I just want to snap her head off.

You can start dealing with anger by monitoring your insides. For a few minutes try shining light on your anger.

Begin by asking who or what your anger is really about. As you do, remember that anger can be a reactive emotion. In fact, anger often comes as a handmaiden to fear.

We see this in Mark, who enjoyed an evening with Dan at a time when Dan was feeling well and optimistic. They laughed for the first time in weeks, and for a while they forgot all about AIDS. The time was good. But with good times comes the fear of losing them. There's more to lose now and that turns Mark's emotional high into a new low: I forget how to enjoy myself sometimes. What if I forget altogether?

In fact, you can feel more angry even when things go better. You might even feel tempted to pick a fight now and then with the PWCI. That makes the whole situation a little "less good." Then there's not as much to lose. Sound familiar?

It's normal to get angry at such times, and it doesn't help to get angry at yourself for feeling this way. At the same time it helps to really know what's going on: Behind the anger is fear of losing what you cherish, a simple fear of not getting your own way. It's natural to want to stay mad, to pull away for a while.

Unless you recognize this you could end up separated from the PWCI and confused about it. It's common to end up mad for "no good reason," snapping at everyone who crosses your path, strangers and friends alike. And you end up feeling bad about yourself in the bargain.

Remember one thing: Sometimes pulling away for a while is a viable choice. And when it is, do it straightforwardly. Move away with more clarity about what you really feel and with more skill in the way you communicate that feeling. Many caregivers find that with increasing awareness they prefer not to remain angry or afraid.

Application 11: Working With Feelings

Think of the last three times you were angry. Jot down a few details. Who or what were you angry at? What happened just before you got angry? How did you act when you were angry? How did it end?

As you look back, ask yourself what you might have feared at the time you were angry. There's no need to dig deep or probe the past. Keep it simple and stick to the present.

Application 12: Working With Feelings

The next time you're angry remember to look for a source of that anger. If you can't, then at least refuse to judge yourself for getting angry. Just allow yourself to become aware of the anger without judging it.

Next, ask yourself what you want to do. Stay angry and afraid or let go of your fear and anger and get some relief. If you want to let go, then consider some of these strategies:

- Talk to someone about your feelings and ask for help in getting perspective.
- Write about your feelings and get some distance that way.
- Grant yourself a "break" from anger. Release yourself from anger or fear for the next five minutes, five hours or even five days.
- Distract yourself by doing something you enjoy or listing the things you enjoy.
- Allow yourself to lighten up. Repeat slogans that help you lighten up. "Don't sweat the small stuff. And remember, it's all small stuff." "It's not a big deal."

Perhaps you'll discover that you really want to hold onto the anger or fear. It's common for people to feel this way, and that's okay, too. If you want to hold onto the negative feeling, then do so. Stay mad, but do it with a little more awareness about the source of that feeling. When you do get ready, allow it to pass.

The path toward acceptance is a bumpy one and there are many curves along the way. Caregivers move through a host of feelings, frustrations of living with and caring for a PWCI and disappointments over not getting what they want. For Mark, the act of accepting Dan's need *not* to tell Tommy and Jay helped Dan feel more comfortable with Mark going out with friends. And the next week, much to Mark's surprise, Dan told their friends that he had AIDS.

3 CONNECTING:

Make Contact With Other People And Yourself

For many people who find themselves in a caregiver role, *connection* provides meaning in their lives. Even before the PWCI got sick, they experienced their happiest times — their sense of completeness and wholeness — *in connection* to others.

This does not necessarily mean they were "in love" with that "special someone." Rather the caregiver made contact with another — or others — mind to mind, heart to heart, soul to soul.

Connection happens for many caregivers in a variety of different ways. It entails dropping the barriers between themselves and others, the defenses that they employ to keep them "safe" and separate from others. Of course, for many people these defenses, instead of keeping them safe, isolate them from the very connections they desire.

This is another one of the paradoxes of human behavior: The "safer" people are, the more isolated and the less fulfilled they are as humans. This is the way it is with many human defenses that become distorted in the process of defending ourselves. When chronic illness enters a person's life, the connection to a loved one is threatened, disrupted and altered.

STELLA, LOLA AND CHRISTINE

Lola had just spent a good part of Saturday at Stella's cleaning, changing linens, doing laundry and cooking meat loaf and apple pie for supper. She worked like a team of sled dogs, racing to finish before Stella and Ted returned from Christine's physical therapy. It pleased both Lola and Stella when Ted accompanied his wife and daughter to the physical therapy sessions because it meant Ted and Stella would be able to talk to other caregivers of people with muscular dystrophy.

It also meant that Ted would not be underfoot when Lola cleaned, and it meant that he'd be somewhat sober, showing some interest in his family.

After dinner Ted settled in front of the TV and began to drink. Lola, Stella and Christine sat at the kitchen table playing rummy. Stella shared with Lola an emotional therapy technique she had learned that day from the social worker while Christine was in physical therapy. The exercise involved writing down changes in relationships that had occurred since becoming involved in the caregiving process. Since Lola was certainly a caregiver, too, Stella encouraged her to participate. The women wrote as they verbalized:

I've learned to appreciate my children more, especially my beautiful Christine. Christine had been such a help at one time, baby-sitting, cleaning, cooking, never complaining, and I never showed my appreciation because I just took her for granted. She enabled me to get out of the house and now I am grounded, but I have no resentment toward

her. Now I must not only take care of little Irene but Christine as well.
My helper needs help. I am spending more time with the children
because I want to make up for lost time. Ted is content watching TV
with his six or twelve pack. He and I don't spend any quality time
together and a part of me says that's okay.

Lola observed that both she and Stella have become more
playful with Christine or at least more involved with her
play since Christine's only playmate Dorothea moved out of
the building with her parents. Lola noted that she was spending at least two more nights a week with Stella, Christine
and Irene and that she and Stella had grown even closer.

Stella admitted she felt guilty about consuming so much
of Lola's time, thinking that it impinged on her potential
social life. "My calendar isn't exactly crammed with party
invitations or dates for the opera, Stella," Lola said. "But the
few friends I have at work and at NA know about Christine
and all the work involved with monitoring Irene and always
show concern. They say they admire me for being so willing
to help you and so willing to give up the bowling league. I
think most of the people on the team are glad I quit. I was
the worst bowler on the team," Lola admitted.

Stella pointed out that even though Lola was a lousy bowler
she was always the member who was the most fun. "You
always made them laugh. Remember when you threw your
ball into the next lane? Or the night you split your stretch
pants right up the seam? I was with you when you bought
those pants. You asked me how you looked in them. I told you
that you looked like a woman going forth in sin. Each cheek
was its own boss, Lola." The women convulsed with laughter,
with Christine joining in, not really understanding some of
the reason for the laughs but grateful to be included.

Lola observed how much fun she and Stella had when
they reminisced and suggested that Christine think of funny
things that had happened to her, her mom or Lola. Lola said
that they must be written down.

DISCOVER YOUR PRESENT
SOURCES OF SUPPORT

As with every other skill explained in this book connecting entails telling the truth about your life as it's happening right now — today. The following applications aim to help you discover your present sources of emotional support. As with any of the applications you can write your responses in a journal. (See Chapter 5 for more help with journaling.) Or you can dictate your responses into a hand-held cassette recorder.

Application 13: Learning

Describe any changes in your significant relationships that you've experienced since you began caring for a PWCI. Do you see family members and close friends less? When you see these people, do you talk about your caregiving experiences? Do you focus on caregiving or do you talk about other subjects as well? Do you still feel close to these people?

Application 14: Learning

Map out the emotional connections to people in your life. One method for doing this is the Attneave Family Network Map developed by Dr. Carolyn L. Attneave of the Boston Family Institute. This map charts family relationships differently than a traditional family tree, which depicts only legal and blood relationships. The purpose of the Family Network Map is to depict how you feel about the various people in your life, including friends and neighbors as well as relatives. To build this map, you first need to make four lists of people:

1. List the names of everyone living in your home. Put yourself down first. Draw a square next to male names and a circle next to female names. If pets are an important part of your life, put a triangle after their names. Then put a 1 in the circle or square for your own name. Then number the remaining names on your list, beginning with the number 2. This list is called your "Zone 1" relationships.

2. List the names of people who are emotionally significant to you. These are people you feel strongly about and see or talk to often. Again, draw a circle or square after each name and number each name. Be sure to include people you strongly dislike or who dislike you, as well as those people you strongly like. (You can add other names to this later and number them as needed. Don't worry if the numbers get out of order on the page.) This list is called your "Zone 2" relationships.

3. List the names of people with whom you have a casual relationship. These are people you feel less strongly about. Number the circles or squares as you did with the previous lists. This list is called your "Zone 3" relationships.

4. Now list people who live far away from you and people you seldom see except on special occasions such as reunions, weddings or funerals. Number their names as you did on the earlier lists. This list is called your "Zone 4" relationships.

Now turn to the Family Network Map on page 38. This is a series of four concentric circles, each circle representing the lists (zones) you just made.

Your next task is to transfer your lists to the map, using just the numbered circle or square for each person. (Do not write anyone's name.) Begin by putting your own number in the center of the circle.

Notice that the right side of the map is for nonfamily members and the left side is for family members. A triangle at the bottom of the map defines a space for listing people you dislike or have difficulty with. These can be family members or nonfamily members.

After you've placed every name from your lists onto the map, draw lines to connect people who know one another. You don't need to draw lines connecting anyone with yourself. The lines will cross each other, similar to the example shown on the next page.

FAMILY NETWORK MAP

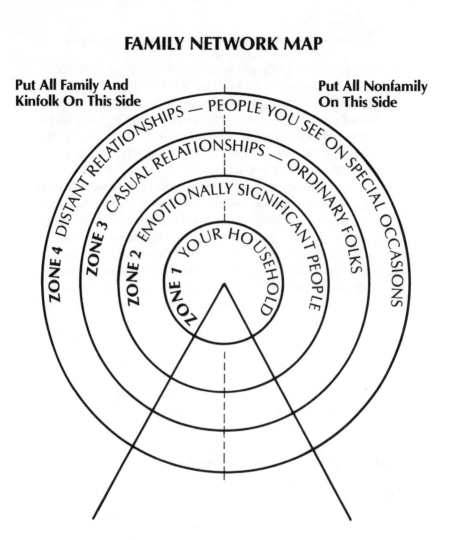

Put All Family And Kinfolk On This Side

Put All Nonfamily On This Side

ZONE 4 DISTANT RELATIONSHIPS — PEOPLE YOU SEE ON SPECIAL OCCASIONS

ZONE 3 CASUAL RELATIONSHIPS — ORDINARY FOLKS

ZONE 2 EMOTIONALLY SIGNIFICANT PEOPLE

ZONE 1 YOUR HOUSEHOLD

Put Any People Who Make You Uncomfortable Or Whom You Dislike Between These Lines

Now consider your map, using the following suggestions:

- You might find someone who connects with a number of people in several zones. Each person is a "nexus" for information and action. What would happen if they moved, died or became ill? Who would take their places? What changes would occur in your life? Do your nexus names include people you dislike? Which zones do they fall in?
- You may also find a small group of several people who know each other and many others on your map. This is a "plexus" in your map — a kind of switchboard for getting information or organizing activity. If your plexus changes, there could be a significant or difficult transition in your life.
- See if there are any "cliques" on your map. A clique is a plexus that is closed — it has no relationship with others.
- Look for any people who seem unconnected. These people may be an important balance for any nexus or plexus in your life. They may share a part of your life that others do not. These people should remain in your life even if a plexus or nexus breaks up.
- Also look at several other features of your map: How many males are present? How many females? What zones have the most people? Are there many people you dislike compared to those you like? Are these family members or non-family members? How has caring for a person with a chronic illness changed your map? (In other words, how would your map look if you'd drawn it before you became a caregiver?)

Now take a moment to construct an "ideal" map. This does not have to include everyone on your first map. What changes would you like to make in your network of relationships? What relationships deserve extra attention right now? Based on what you've discovered, write a goal that describes change you'd like to make in one of your relationships. Then list two or three concrete actions you can take toward this goal.

Application 15: Learning

List the sources of emotional support in your life, the type of support they offer and how much support comes from each source. Include people in your list, but also include places that you find relaxing or regenerating as well as activities that calm or renew you.

Now look over your list. Are you receiving all the emotional support you want or need? If your answer is no, then choose one concrete action you can take in the next week to bring another source of emotional support into your life. Consider joining a caregivers support group, calling a social service agency for respite care or making a standing monthly appointment to eat dinner with a friend you haven't seen much since you became a primary caregiver.

Application 16: Learning

Have changes taken place in your work relationship because of caring for a person with chronic illness? Describe them.

After describing any changes that have taken place in your work situation and key relationships, evaluate these developments. Do you see the changes as positive or negative? Would you like your present work situation or work-related relationships to change in any way? How?

Choose one change you'd like to make and list one specific task you could take toward making that change. For example, you could make arrangements to work at home one day a week so that you have more flexibility to balance your work and caregiving tasks.

Application 17: Taking Action

It's easy for caregivers to lose contact with friends. One strategy is to make a weekly or monthly appointment to see close friends. Give this appointment the same priority you'd give to a medical appointment or a business meeting.

Right now, think of someone you could contact. Write down this person's name and phone number.

Next, make plans to see this person or talk over the phone. It helps to be specific. On what date will you do this? If you plan to meet in person, where will you meet and when? Note the date and time on your calendar.

Consider making such a "connection appointment" at least once every month. Begin by adding to your list of names and phone numbers now.

JOIN A CAREGIVERS SUPPORT GROUP
AND SEEK COUNSELING

An excellent way to expand your circle of support is to join a support group for caregivers. In such a group, you'll meet other caregivers who have had similar experiences and feelings. Because these people know caregiving first-hand, they'll be able to listen and understand you like few others can. In these groups the basis for connection is the common ground on which you walk. This can be a heartening experience for many caregivers.

How do you find such a group? Here are a few places to start:

- Social service agencies
- Churches and synagogues
- Public health services
- Hospitals
- YMCAs and YWCAs
- Mental health agencies
- Associations that focus on certain conditions (such as the Muscular Dystrophy Society, the American Cancer Sociey or the American Diabetes Association). Look for local branches of these associations in your community.

You can also call the National Self-Help Clearinghouse, (212) 642-2944. Ask if there are any support groups for caregivers in your area. There is also a list of agencies in the back of this book.

Finding an existing group is often the easiest route to take at first. In some cases, the agencies you contact may not know of one. If this happens, suggest that they start a caregivers support group and consider helping them do so.

If you want a support group to work for you, here are some suggestions:

- Admit that you have a problem and accept it.

- Be willing to support other people who share your problem.
- Speak openly. Tell your story. Share thoughts and feelings that you'd normally withhold. An effective group is a safe nonthreatening place.
- Listen with an open mind. Before you comment on what other people say, take time to hear them, to understand them. Be willing to learn from others.
- Accept help from other people. Remember that "you alone can do it, but you can't do it alone."
- Set clear goals for yourself and ask other group members for help in reaching those goals. Describe a specific problem you face, then listen to how other group members have solved that problem.

A skilled group leader — someone you trust — is one of the keys to a successful group. Such a person keeps the group discussion on track without forcing it down a certain path. A good leader also ensures that everyone who wants to speak gets a chance to do so, prompts people to speak clearly and openly, and helps group members resolve conflict.

One of the most healing aspects of a support group is that caregivers discover they are not alone. What they feel, others also feel. What they think, others think. Caregivers in these groups find out that others have struggled with the same day-to-day issues and survived. Caregivers experience a blend of identification with others, as well as a sense that other caregivers have different experiences, too. Connection emerges from the similarities, from appreciation of differences, as well as from a sense of caring for other group members.

Some people who join a support group for the first time feel awkward when the attention of the group is focused on them. Some caregivers don't feel their issues are "important" enough for such consideration. Remember: You deserve this support. You are worthy of this attention. The work you do as a caregiver is important, not only to your family but to society.

It's possible that you might experience some negative feelings after joining a group. For a time you might feel slightly worse than before. If that happens, don't give up on the group right away. Try to determine the source of those negative feelings. Do they come from the fact that you're confronting some painful issues for the first time? Or do they spring from something you feel about a certain person in the group? Attend at least a month's worth of meetings before you answer this question. Try and identify what is upsetting to you and develop a plan to work through it.

Caregivers may also benefit greatly from seeing a counselor privately. There you can talk about an issue that's not fully addressed in your support group, and you can talk about any problems you're having with the group itself. A counselor can also give you detailed help in learning a specific skill, such as how to set limits or speak assertively. Connections made with a professional counselor or therapist (or caregiver) are important for many people who provide care to others.

CONNECT TO OTHER CAREGIVERS
IN YOUR FAMILY

Chronic illness stresses the whole family system — even when one family member assumes primary responsibility for caregiving. In addition, this stress can intensify old family roles and conflicts as we've seen with Rose and Paul.

In many families, for example, it's just assumed that one person will take over as primary caregiver while other people are free of such family "responsibilities." Sometimes family members are frightened by the illness; others see it as their duty to take control; still others may become compulsive about caregiving tasks as a way to avoid their own pain;

and some family members may in effect disappear, that is, stay out of emotional contact altogether.

Such family roles are often discussed in a negative way. But it's important not to condemn them. Such roles are often forged during times of stress, and they are one way for caregivers to deal with the chaos chronic illness brings to their lives. These behaviors may have made sense in the past, but they may not today.

Family roles often lead to conflict, and that can be especially hard on caregivers. Family conflict saps energy — energy that's needed for going about their lives — living, working, playing and caregiving.

There's a hidden gift in family tension, however. While it's not easy to live with, chronic illness usually brings family issues to the forefront. It brings those issues to the surface and throws them in sharp relief. That focus and clarity can make it easier to see what needs to be done. It can also enhance the conflict.

The solution is not to abandon roles — it's to choose your roles and to be free of any that don't serve you. Family conflicts can be worked out when people become flexible, when they're willing to take on new behaviors in response to chronic illness. And anything you can do to lessen family conflict overall will make your job as caregiver easier.

First, remember you have the choice as a caregiver to share your pain and ask for help, especially from family members. Even though caregivers often know they could turn to others, they don't. They still act as if they're somehow obligated to work in isolation. This, too, can go back to old, unquestioned family patterns.

For example, in Rita's family, Pearl is the caregiver. She always has been and always will be. And she feels unable to ask for help from Rita. Both are isolated from each other and need each other all the more.

Be in direct communication with all family members. Families in distress often abound in triangles. Two people in conflict with each other do not share their thoughts and feelings directly with each other. Instead they complain to a third party. In the case of Mark and Phyllis both complain to Dan, the identified patient. Ironically this puts a strain on the family and the process of caregiving, and increases the stress for the PWCI.

You can break this cycle. Someone in your family may be locked in unresolved conflict with another family member, constantly expressing ill feelings that are never revealed directly to the person concerned. When this person is with you, try starting with, "Let's just talk about us." This is a reasonable request that seems intuitively right. And through this simple statement you can weaken the triangle. You can encourage family members to deal directly with the person with whom they are in conflict and not provide an outlet for them to complain about someone else.

Consider asking for a family conference to talk about caregiving tasks. You need not call it by this name. Especially in families where chronic illness is an "open secret" (something that people know but never discuss), simply speaking openly about your concerns is a place to start. And if you cannot speak to everyone concerned at once, then speak to a few people. Sometimes powerful family conferences take place between just two people at a time.

If your family does gather as a group, then remember the following:

- Consider asking a neutral person to attend as a kind of "moderator." This person could be a family friend, a counselor, a priest, minister or rabbi. An effective moderator, not being a family member, can have a cooler, more detached perspective on emotionally charged issues. This person's job is to make sure everyone is heard and to keep the discussion on issues and not on personalities.
- Start with a simple expectancy of possible outcomes. The goal is to open lines of communication rather

than expect that everyone will resolve their issues, kiss and make up.

- Let everyone speak. Even more than agreement, family members simply want to be heard. Before you respond to what another person says, sum up what you think that person said. Then ask if you got it right.
- When you tread on highly emotional ground, talk first about what you see — the objective events that others can observe also. For example, instead of saying, "You always run away when Mom gets sick," try "Whenever Mom goes into the hospital, I don't know where you are or how to reach you." After stating what you observe, then you can discuss how you feel about it. As much as possible stick to "I" messages. (See pages 58-59.) "When I can't reach you, I get scared about what would happen if she died."
- Plan for the future. Anticipate what the person with chronic illness will need tomorrow, next week or next year. Avoid family conferences that just rehash the past. Instead, focus on the future and remind everyone that the aim is to help the person with chronic illness. That can take the spotlight off old family battles. Focus on an action.
- Give your family time to heal. It's unlikely that after years deeply ingrained roles will change overnight. Some family members may even resent your attempts to change the status quo and emotionally dig in their heels. That's okay. Remember that their reactions are beyond your control and keep asking these people to say what they're thinking and feeling. Listen without judging. Be willing to walk away, even if you don't get what you want.

Application 18: Learning

For the next week pay attention to your conversations with and about family members. How many of these conversations focus on saying negative things about people who are not present to the conversation?

Now decide what you want to do with the results of this exercise. Are there other things you can talk about when conversations get negative? What can you say or do that will bring a positive influence to the situation? Write down a few simple ideas.

Application 19: Taking Action

Imagine you're going to hold a family conference tonight. Who do you want to show up? What do you want on the agenda? Write down a list of participants and a tentative agenda. Get input from other family members.

When you're done, strongly consider holding this conference, even if you decide not to discuss everything on your agenda or invite everyone you've listed. Schedule a time and choose a moderator/facilitator.

Following is what happened to Rose as she did this exercise.

ROSE, ELSIE AND MICHAEL

Rose detailed in her notebook plans for the family conference, as Dr. Wilburforce suggested. It would have to be on neutral turf and at a convenient time — during her and John's annual winter soak in Miami. The day before the holidays probably would suit everyone since businesses would be tightly shuttered and people would be in a holiday mood. The place for the conference would be the balcony of her parent's condo, overlooking the ocean to one side and the coast highway on the other side. The Atlantic would look rehearsed. She would have it catered. But could she find a caterer on such short notice? Perhaps just cold cuts, John's favorite.

Her insightful daughter, Lisa, and the baby would be in from Syracuse. She wondered if her son-in-law Joel could get away. He would be the voice of impartial reason. John would wear one of his pastel outfits, looking like some toothpick sucker on his way to a Pebble Beach Open.

On the other hand, Paul would be dressed more formally. Oh, she'd have to do something about John's wardrobe. Paul and his bride would be as sensitive as toilet seats. She remembered that line from one of her English lit classes at Barnard — Holden Caufield spoke it, she wrote.

Dr. Wilburforce quickly read the rest of Rose's entry: Why Brandon would remain in New York, what excuse she'd offer, what she'd wear, how she'd greet her brother — a kiss or a handshake?

He put down Rose's notebook. "Rose, are you writing a novel or planning a family conference? It's good and healthy to write in stream of consciousness, but this was not the assignment. It's a good start, but you avoided the unpleasant issues: (1) Telling your father the purpose of the family conference, (2) Confronting Paul and letting him know you feel he has to start shouldering some of the responsibility, (3) Telling John that you might have to spend months at a time away from him and Brandon, and (4) Getting your folks to buy the idea of a nursing home and handling the actual last day when your parents walk out of their home."

Rose saw that she was indeed, as usual, avoiding the unpleasant issues and affirmed that she'd rework the assignment. "Oh, Doctor," Rose said, "I remember a time when all I had to worry about was whether John's cold cuts were fresh and his collars starched!"

CONNECT TO COMMUNITY SERVICES

When people think about connecting, the first thoughts that usually come to mind are about connecting with friends, other family members and a support group. The list does not have to stop there, however. Consider community services, too.

Several trends in American society are waking people to the needs of caregivers. One is the fact that, thanks to new therapies and medical technology, people are living longer. At the same time, living longer does not always mean living in good health. Millions of older adults depend on friends, family members or nursing homes for full- or part-time care. Add to this another fact: More and more of this country's health-care dollars are going to pay for the effects of chronic illness. The major killers in this culture have shifted from acute diseases and infections to chronic conditions such as heart disease and cancer, diseases that are deeply influenced by personal choice and lifestyle.

There is a growing network of community services. In fact, special services exist with the caregiver in mind. Start with the nearest county social service agency, public health agency or chapter of the United Way. Some of the programs you may discover are the following:

- **Adult day care.** Programs that provide professional caregivers during the day for people with chronic illness or disability, relieving you of some of the responsibility and providing some needed relief.
- **Adult foster care.** Supervised care in licensed homes for people who can no longer live independently.
- **Companions or "buddies."** People who will come into your home and help with meals, cleaning, shopping and personal care for people with chronic illness.
- **Home-delivered meals.** Services, such as the federally-sponsored Meals-on-Wheels, that prepare and deliver food directly to the home.
- **Homemaking assistance.** Supervised and trained people who can help with cleaning, shopping and other household tasks.
- **Home health care.** In-home assistance with bathing, toileting, eating and mobility for people with chronic illness or disability. Certified home health agencies employ trained people, usually supervised by a registered nurse.

- **Visitor services.** Regular calls or visits to homebound people. Formal visitor services are usually supervised by social workers.
- **Counseling.** Help with the emotional impact of chronic illness, both for the person with illness and caregivers as well. Often counseling includes work on specific skills: managing stress, asking for what you want, making decisions, setting goals, managing time, managing money and the like.
- **Chore services.** Services that help with yard work, snow removal, heavy cleaning and other home maintenance.
- **Respite care.** Secondary caregivers who give primary caregivers a "break." Sometimes these people come into the home for a limited time; in other cases the person with chronic illness may go to a nursing home, hospital or residential care center for a short time.
- **Transportation services.** They provide travel to and from medical appointments and other community services.

This is just a partial list. Your area may offer more services. Also note that the names of such programs differ across communities. Just describe in general the service you want or the need you'd like to have filled. That should help you get connected to an appropriate service.

Application 20: Taking Action

Make a list of basic daily needs as they relate to your caregiving role. What tasks might you get help with? Where might you find help in your community? Look up at least one number to call and inquire about the availability and costs of such help.

CONNECT TO THE WORLD

In *Religions of Man*, Huston Smith sums up the basic perspective of the world's religions in a single insight: "The self is too small an object for perpetual enthusiasm." Poet John Donne echoed the idea with the line, "No man is an island, entire of itself; every man is a piece of the continent, a part of the main."

Life is filled with opportunities to grow beyond oneself, to enlarge one's sphere of concern so that it grows beyond the confines of individual likes and dislikes, daily disappointments and triumphs. People grow by thinking bigger, by bringing to life something that is larger and more enduring than themselves. This idea may seem redundant in a book about caregiving. Are not caregivers already intimately involved with other people's needs? Are they not already connected, serving others and forgetting themselves for many hours each day?

Caregivers find themselves in an emotionally charged situation — one in which their needs and the needs of PWCIs are intertwined. Sometimes, in fact, they can get so mixed up that their moods depend entirely on the moods of the PWCIs. Mark, upon waking in the morning, asks Dan, "How am I feeling today?"

Sometimes caregiving can make caregivers "smaller." Instead of helping them see the pettiness and impermanence of most of their worries, it can give them more worries, more emotional ups and downs — those of their PWCIs. Instead of growing beyond themselves and connecting to the larger human community, they can forget the outside world even exists. Instead of truly serving, they shrink.

People with chronic illness can benefit from making their world larger. The PWCIs can become caregivers themselves. The person who is HIV positive and still active can become a buddy to someone with AIDS. The person with multiple sclerosis can start a support group for other people with neurological conditions. The person with diabetes can help teach other diabetics how to maintain their health. One recovering alcoholic sustains his or her sobriety by working with other alcoholics.

As a caregiver you can encourage PWCIs to feel a part of events in their families, their communities, their world. When appropriate, suggest that they become actively involved in volunteer work. Tasks such as writing letters, making phone calls and typing or dictating can be done at home by people with limited mobility. Even with the limits on activity that a chronic illness imposes, people can often take actions that make them "larger" — that connect them with the outside world.

When people connect in this way, they glimpse the deeper meaning of caring. "Caring," as philosopher Milton Mayeroff explains, "is helping anything or anyone come to life, to grow from idea to reality." In this sense you can care for ideas and projects as well as people. The person who starts a rape crisis center, the person who writes a book, the person who volunteers in an elementary school — all of them are caring in this larger sense. And it's to this level of caring that all people — including people with chronic illness — can aspire.

GET OUT THE NEWS
WITHOUT DRAINING YOURSELF

One of the most frequent tasks caregivers face is providing information and updates about PWCIs. Family members, friends, insurance companies, health-care providers, all of them monitor the health of PWCIs. And as primary caregiver, they may turn to you for that information.

If you find yourself repeating the same information time and time again to different people, it can have some subtle effects and it can be tiring. You may end up feeling like the focus is always on the PWCI — not on you or what you need to maintain your own sanity.

Much of this chapter has been about expanding your sources of support. An excellent way to involve your widening circle of support is to have them help get out the news. Here are some strategies:

- Ask two or three people to be contacts that other people can call with questions about the PWCI. Inform these people about any significant changes in the health of the PWCI.
- Enlist others to be patient advocates for the PWCI. These people go by different names: sponsor, buddy, advisor or friend. These people can listen to medical reports, take notes, ask questions and tell others.
- Encourage people who want to know about the PWCI to speak directly with that person if it's possible.
- Make sure you can still connect with friends who are important to you on levels other than those about illness.

DON'T WAIT — CREATE

One of your primary challenges as a caregiver is to cease feeling like a victim. Instead of waiting for bad news, you can make your own news. Instead of waiting for someone else to give you directions, you can choose what actions you'll take. In short, you can act instead of waiting to be acted upon.

One of the ways to do so is to connect with your own creativity. It's important to realize that the term "creative" does not just apply to musicians, painters, poets and dancers. Everyone is creative. After all, creativity is bringing something into being that did not exist before — or combining things that already exist in a new way.

The person who writes a letter creates ideas. The teacher creates an environment for learning. The computer programmer creates a set of instructions that directs a computer to perform a certain task. The friend who listens well creates an atmosphere of trust and acceptance. Anyone who solves a problem is creative and, in that sense, caregivers are creating all the time!

"Rather than wait for bad news, we create," said Mark. "And that doesn't have to mean creating a timeless work of art. Dan and I can do a crossword puzzle together or build a card house. We grow plants together. We draw castles together or paint each other's portraits (although none will ever hang in the Louvre). We weave fantasies together, we dream together. It beats sitting around all day and complaining about how lousy he or I feel."

Creativity may even enhance human immune systems in a way that can make people more healthy. In his book *Anatomy of an Illness*, Norman Cousins wrote about his meeting with Pablo Casals, the cellist, and one of the great musicians of the twentieth century. This meeting took place shortly before Casals' ninetieth birthday, when the musician's health was not ideal. He had emphysema and breathed in a labored way. He also had arthritis, walked with a shuffle and needed help dressing. Yet Casals still played music daily, including a practice session at the piano.

Cousins was present one day when Casals arranged himself, with great difficulty, at the piano. When Casals started playing, a miracle took place. His hands, which were swollen and clenched, became more supple and flexible. "The fingers slowly unlocked and reached toward the keys like the buds of a plant toward the sunlight," observed Cousins. "His back straightened. He seemed to breathe more freely."

Cousins watched while Casals began playing Bach's "Wohltemperierte Klavier," then a Brahms concerto. "His entire body became fused with the music," Cousins wrote. "It was no longer stiff and shrunken, but supple and graceful and completely freed of its arthritic coils." After he finished practicing, Casals looked and moved in a new way. He stood straighter; he walked without a shuffle. And after eating a hearty breakfast, he went for a long walk on the beach near his home.

Being creative may not alter your health, or the health of those you care for, as dramatically as Casals' creativity did. But creative activity can help you lose yourself for a while. It draws on a different part of yourself than the one used in daily caregiving and provides opportunities to be constructive. When you create, you experiment, you play in the best sense of the word. In short, creativity delivers all the pleasure of doing work that you care passionately about. Each of these qualities makes creativity a healing force in your life.

Application 21: Taking Action

What creative activities do you enjoy? List them. As you make this list, keep your mind open to many possibilities. Anything from sewing to poetry, gardening, skiing, reading, music or sports, as long as it's something you enjoy. Add activities you might like to try that you've never done before.

Now look over the list you just made. Have you stopped doing any of these activities since you started caring for a PWCI? Circle those.

Next, ask yourself if you could resume any of the activities you just circled. Or could you begin any of the other activities on the list?

Choose one activity and list two or three simple steps you could take within the next week to enjoy that activity. For example, if you like to draw, plan to browse in an art supply store and perhaps get a sketch pad and some new pencils.

The following vignette shows how this application played out for Stella, Lola and Christine.

STELLA, LOLA AND CHRISTINE

On the subway ride home from Stella's that Saturday night, Lola reflected on the written exercise she and Stella had done and just how much she missed bowling nights and league involvement. Practically her entire life besides work, sleep and a weekly NA meeting centered around helping Stella care for Christine, Irene and their apartment. She also lent a strong shoulder and compliant ear whenever Stella needed help because of Ted's drinking and neglect. Although Lola enjoyed her caregiver's role and recognized that it had become part of her, like the butterfly tattooed on her left hip, it was becoming clearer to her that four nights and one entire weekend day might be too much time to spend at caregiving. She needed some "me time" and she also recognized that Stella needed "me time," too.

She couldn't wait to get back to her apartment to phone Stella. They would *both* join a bowling team. Lola would call around on Monday to see what leagues were forming. Stella would call the Muscular Dystrophy Association and the Childhood Diabetes Association to see what sorts of evening home care were available to spell beleaguered caregivers. Both women agreed that Ted could not be counted on to be at home, sober or conscientious enough to administer insulin to Irene and monitor the girls.

Lola and Stella agreed they were in a rut and that their lives were stagnant. "We won't feel so stale and trapped and God knows I could use the exercise," said Lola. "Our getting out will also help Christine. She needs different companionship besides you and me. This is going to work out fine, Stella," she bubbled.

Lola urged Stella to make a list of all the fun things she used to do before Irene was born and before Christine was diagnosed with muscular dystrophy. She and Stella would go over the list on Monday and work out a way to engage in some of those fun activities again.

TURN COMPLAINTS INTO SOLUTIONS

Caregivers commonly experience complaints. Some complain about never having enough time, about feeling tired and drained, about not knowing what the future will bring. What's more, caregivers find themselves listening to complaints from the PWCI — complaints about physicians who don't respond, about medications that bring side effects, about pain or about other symptoms. Internalizing negative thoughts and feelings is one of the prime ways caregivers exhaust themselves. They absorb negative energy and drain themselves via complaining.

You can start to change this situation by looking at complaints in a new way. Instead of being a source of irritation, complaints can be a source of information. Instead of posing problems, they can point to solutions. "I'm always confused about my illness" can become "Please help me understand what my doctor is telling me." "I'm feeling trapped by this illness" can become "Help me find new friends and new things to do, even when I don't feel good."

This viewpoint is common to almost every method of resolving conflict. For example, in his book *Getting To Yes*, Roger Fisher outlines four steps for resolving conflict:

- Separate the person from the problem.
- Focus on interests, not positions.
- Develop options for mutual gain.
- Insist on objective criteria.

In the application that follows you'll use a modified version of these steps.

Application 22: Taking Action

The purpose of this exercise is to help you turn complaints into solutions. Picture yourself as the manager of a complaint department — you're the boss and you have the answers. You are wise and competent.

First, write down the complaint in one sentence. For example, "He never lets me have time alone, even when he's feeling good."

Now rewrite the complaint as a problem statement or request. Be kind, clear and firm. Example: "I'd like to spend a little more time alone."

Next, brainstorm solutions to the problem: "When I want some time alone, I'll leave a note on the kitchen table or schedule some time alone and get 'coverage' from my job as caregiver so I can engage in a fun activity." Let the PWCI know in advance. "I care for you and I'd like some time alone to do gardening. So next week Brenda will hang out here while I go to a flower show." Finally, choose three effective solutions and follow up on them. Choose one simple action you could take immediately to resolve the problem or follow up on the request. For example,

"I'd like to get outside for a walk today. How about if I do that while you're napping?"

COMMUNICATION — TAKING RESPONSIBILITY

It will be helpful if you can learn to take responsibility for the quality of your emotional life, no matter how many distressing events you face on a daily basis. This notion of responsibility — or the lack of it — is echoed in language. There's a world of difference between "You make me feel sad" and "When you're sick, I feel sad."

These two statements illustrate the difference between "I" and "you" messages. "I" statements let you take responsibility for what you're feeling. "You" statements blame other people and put them on the defensive. Knowing the difference between these two kinds of messages is a key to the art of assertiveness, the subject of so many books and seminars over the past 20 years.

Here are some more examples of "you" statements:

- "You never let me get a word in edgewise."
- "Being around you all the time makes me tired."
- "You're irresponsible and never show up on time."

Below are some examples of those "you" statements rephrased as "I" statements:

- "When we talk, I find it hard to finish a sentence."
- "During the last month, I've had a lot less energy."
- "I went to pick you up at the airport and ended up waiting two hours. I didn't know where you were."

An effective "I" statement includes at least one of the following elements:

- What I observe.
- What I feel.
- What I think.

- What I want.
- What I intend to do.

Effective "I" statements are specific rather than general.
You can take an example from Pearl asking Rita's physician questions about a new medication as part of Rita's chemotherapy.

- "I notice that when I ask you a question, you don't look at me." (What I observe.)
- "When I get confused, I feel anxious." (What I feel.)
- "When I ask you a question, I listen to the answer and still end up confused." (What I think.)
- "I would like to make sure I understand this treatment so I can be helpful when it is administered." (What I want.)
- "If I cannot get my questions answered, I'm going to ask for a second opinion." (What I intend to do.)

This whole issue of assertiveness applies directly to people who seek medical care for chronic illness. Dr. Bernie Seigel, a surgeon and author of *Love, Medicine and Miracles*, urges people with chronic illness not to be "good patients" — especially when that means following orders and keeping their mouths shut. However, the alternative to being a "good patient" is not blaming and attacking — being a "bad patient." "I" messages can help you get your point across without blame or judgment. It's health-promoting to participate in the health-care process with professional caregivers. Ask questions, express opinions and wishes. Collaborate.

Changing "you" statements into "I" statements is one of the most powerful communication skills you can learn. Gaining this skill can help you resolve conflict, reduce tension and manage the stress that sometimes comes when you feel powerless to help the PWCI.

Keep in mind that you may run into resistance when you use "I" messages to speak assertively. This can happen, for example, with family members or professional caregivers (doctors, nurses) who are not used to this type of communication. Some of them may resent any attempt to change the status quo of unspoken rules and "open secrets." They may be surprised — even shocked — if you announce what you think, what you feel, what you want and what you intend to do.

That reaction makes sense; after all, they're used to you behaving a certain way. You can help people adjust to assertive communication by explaining why you're using "I" messages. Point out that your aim is to resolve conflict and keep the focus off personalities. Most of all, you want to ensure that you and the PWCI live in an atmosphere of openness, trust and love.

Being assertive takes energy, sometimes lots of energy. Use this skill in relationships where it matters the most. This means "picking your battles" and letting go of minor irritations. It's important to be assertive with your medical team and the PWCI. You might practice being assertive with the repair person who shows up at your house 30 minutes late or with the mail carrier who accidentally delivers a package meant for you to the neighbor across the street. Practice using "I" messages for situations where it doesn't make much difference to your peace of mind in the long run so that when it matters, you'll be better able to apply these techniques in a more natural fashion.

Application 23: Taking Action

Write an "I" message that you can use when talking to the PWCI. Include at least one of these elements: what you observe, what you feel, what you think, what you want or what you intend to do. Make your statement in a way that does not cast blame on the person to whom you're talking. For example, Stella can assert, "I want you to stop drinking. I feel awful when you come home drunk, Ted. The kids don't like to be around you when you're that way. If you're drunk, it would be better for us if you slept elsewhere until you sober up. Someday, I hope you'll stop drinking for good."

Application 24: Taking Action

Write an assertive "no" statement — a statement that you could use in actual conversation. Use an "I" message as the core of your statement. For example, Stella can tell Ted, "I will no longer cook you a meal if you are drunk — and I certainly won't sleep with you."

Connecting with the PWCI can be a great source of solace in the face of illness. Caregiving is a comprehensive task, requiring compassion, availability, strength and consistency. Caregivers need to care for themselves and replenish their energies so they will be able to carry on better. Healthy caregiving means connecting while maintaining a sense of oneself, thus promoting balance in this difficult yet rewarding job.

4 RELATING:

Gain Intimacy And Balance In Relationships

Healthy relationships between caregivers and PWCIs evolve gradually. These relationships involve movement — both toward and away from each other. This chapter will explore some of the many ways in which caregivers establish intimacy and healthy distance.

GETTING PAST CO-DEPENDENT BEHAVIOR

In any discussion of caregiving it is helpful to include the subject of co-dependence. A brief look at the history of the term sheds some light on how co-dependence applies to caregiving.

Co-dependence originally comes from the literature on alcoholism. It applies to a person in the alcoholic's family who plays a key role in enabling the alcoholic to continue drinking. Often this is the alcoholic's spouse. For instance, the spouse would "cover" when the alcoholic's drinking got out of hand: If the alcoholic husband was too hung over to go to work, then his wife would call in sick for him. Or if the alcoholic wife passed out from a drinking binge, her husband would tell the children, "Mom is sick and can't be with us tonight."

This situation leads to using certain defense mechanisms. One is denial. This happens when the alcoholic's loved ones pretend there's really no problem. "She can quit drinking anytime." "He gets to work almost every day, so there's no way he could be an alcoholic."

Another result is enabling. This means refusing to let the alcoholic experience the consequences of his or her behavior. When the alcoholic's wife calls in sick for her husband, she enables him to avoid a possible consequence (getting fired). And when the alcoholic's husband lies to the children about their mother's drinking, he enables her to avoid a consequence (having to admit openly that she was drunk and couldn't get to the school play).

There's also compulsive caretaking. This happens when covering up the alcoholic's behavior becomes an obsession. For the compulsive caretaker life's central purpose becomes cleaning up messes the alcoholic leaves behind. Often caretakers feel enmeshed with the alcoholic. They cannot feel happy unless the alcoholic is happy. And when the alcoholic is depressed or angry, the caretaker experiences similar emotions or an inverse emotion — guilt and responsibility.

This is an impossible role to fill and the resulting strain can lead to other desperate behaviors. All these behaviors — including denial, enabling and compulsive caretaking — are often called co-dependent behaviors.

In recent years there have been many lists of co-dependent thoughts, feelings and actions in popular self-help books. One of the first appeared in *Adult Children of Alcoholics* by

Janet Woititz. According to Woititz, children who grew up in alcoholic households, among other things, tend to:

- Guess at what normal behavior is.
- Lie when it would be just as easy to tell the truth.
- Over-react to changes over which they have no control.
- Have difficulty with intimate relationships.
- Constantly seek approval.
- Judge themselves without mercy.

Claudia Black, a therapist who works with adult children of alcoholics, pares down the list, saying that children in alcoholic families tend to live out three simple rules: Don't Talk, Don't Trust, Don't Feel.

Another list came from Tony A., a member of the first support group for adult children of alcoholics. (*The Laundry List: The ACoA Experience* by Tony A. with Dan F.) Describing his own experience in an alcoholic family, Tony wrote that:

- We live life from the viewpoint of victims and are attracted by that weakness in our love and friendship relationships.
- We confuse love and pity and tend to "love" people we can "pity" and "rescue."
- We have "stuffed" our feelings from our traumatic childhoods and have lost the ability to feel or express our feelings because it hurts too much.
- We are dependent personalities who are terrified of abandonment, and we will do anything to hold on to a relationship in order not to experience the painful abandonment feelings that we received from living with people who were never emotionally there for us.

Some caregivers look over such lists and see themselves. Co-dependent behaviors, they say, come naturally to them in the effort to care for the PWCI. They, too, feel enmeshed with the PWCI. They may deny that the chronic illness exists, pretend they're fully in control of the PWCI's well-being or believe that they should be in control. Sometimes these care-givers feel they are the reason for a decline in their loved one's health. They feel as if they're walking on eggs to avoid making matters worse. As they experience less control, they try all the more to make things better, which of course is impossible and often makes them feel even worse.

THINK CAREFULLY
ABOUT CO-DEPENDENCE

The word *co-dependence* applies to behaviors, not people. Sometimes people under great stress behave in ways that appear co-dependent, and caregivers typically are under fre-quent stress. This does not mean that the behavior is a per-manent character trait or that these people are co-dependent.

Co-dependence can start sounding a lot like some ideas about sin or being defective. You can use the term to judge yourself harshly, constantly harp on your shortcomings or conclude that you'll never measure up to the ideal of the "perfect" caregiver. In fact, no such caregiver exists. Striving for perfection is admirable though unrealistic. But expecting yourself to be perfect is co-dependent behavior and usually interferes with caregiving.

Learning about co-dependence can give you some helpful pointers. It can help you spot behavior that keeps you un-happy and doesn't serve the PWCI. Don't put the focus on judging or labeling yourself, but on changing the behavior that isn't working for you.

Application 25: Learning

Read the following list of statements. Do any of them "strike home" for you in relating to the PWCI? Write down those that do. Also add any related statements you can think of.

My good feelings about who I am stem from being liked by you.

My good feelings about who I am stem from receiving approval from you.

Your struggles affect my serenity. My mental attention focuses on solving your problems or relieving your pain.

My mental attention is focused on pleasing you.

My mental attention is focused on protecting you.

My mental attention is focused on manipulating you "to do it my way."

My own hobbies and interests aren't important. My time is spent sharing your interests and hobbies.

I am not aware of how I feel; I am aware of how you feel.

I am not aware of what I want; I ask what you want. If you don't tell me, I assume I know what you want.

My social circle diminishes as I involve myself with you.

My fear of your anger determines what I do or say.

My fear of rejection determines what I do or say.

Application 26: Taking Action

Choose a specific alternative to any co-dependent behavior you've seen in yourself. Following is a list to get you started. Again, add any other ideas you have.

- Write your own declaration of independence, spelling out that you want to change any "manipulation without representation" in your life. Then spell out how you intend to change. For example, "I pledge that I will say what I think and feel, even if I take the risk of offending you."
- Arrange a time with the PWCI when you're both feeling calm.
- Explain the co-dependent behaviors that trouble you and how you intend to change them.
- Plan to state what you feel in the very moment that you feel manipulated, hurt or angry. Avoid putting off such statements for a "better" time.
- At a party or family gathering, spend time apart from the PWCI.
- Post a reminder where you'll see it often: "I have no responsibility to make other people happy. Others make themselves happy."
- Promise that you will stop giving orders or taking orders.

• Block out specific times on your calendar for recreation —
for activities you'll do alone or with friends. Share this schedule with the PWCI.

Application 27: Taking Action

Part of becoming a more effective caregiver is forgiving yourself for ineffective behavior. Even the actions you label co-dependent serve a purpose. In order to let go of this behavior it
helps to acknowledge its "payoff."

To begin, list specific co-dependent behaviors in your life.

List what benefit you gain from each behavior. Do they work?
Even if they work sometimes, do they have any hidden costs?
What is the payoff? What are the costs?

Decide if you really want to change these behaviors.

List alternatives to each behavior. Make them specific and
concrete.

Write down any obstacles you feel will prevent you from
practicing the new behavior.

What can you do to get past each obstacle? Write a strategy
to overcome each obstacle.

When Mark did this application, he discovered the following.

DAN AND MARK

Mark listed these co-dependent behaviors:

1. *I feel responsible for Dan's well-being.*
2. *When he is sick and down and depressed, it seems I am down
   and depressed, and when he is up and better, I am in good
   spirits.*

Mark considered the payoff of such co-dependent behavior:

1. *It gives me a sense of power.*
2. *I feel good about myself when I help Dan.*

And he noted the costs:

1. *When Dan feels bad despite all I've done, I feel like a failure. I feel frustrated that I'm so limited.*
2. *The more I do for him, the more dependent he becomes and he grows to expect me to be there for him always. I resent his feeling "entitled" to my attention all the time.*

Mark knew that his behavior was not totally healthy and entered in his journal what he'd like to change, particularly the instances when his moods were dependent on Dan's. Once again he wrote, "When Dan is down, I am down, and he is down too often and for too long." He thought of the line. "We've been down so long even the floor looks like up!" "How sadly applicable," mused Mark. He continued to write.

I am not happy being in a funk. I love him and am deeply concerned, but I must do something to pull myself out of this morass, since I can't do anything more for Dan. Instead of becoming and remaining depressed and fatigued when he's down and feeling exhausted, I can try to predict or anticipate his moods.

I can call the day-care person to find out if Dan's mood is sour, if he's endlessly complaining, if he's fatigued. Or I can phone home and talk to Dan directly and ask him what his energy level is like. I can ask him to anticipate what his energy level will be like in the evening. I can judge his disposition by his response. If I go directly home after work and he's in bed in a darkened room, I'll be more likely to become depressed and tired. However, if I stop off at the gym for an invigorating swim or a forty-five-minute upbeat aerobic workout, I can bring home that upbeat attitude. I'll be better prepared to fight the doom and gloom. There is no need for us to live in a state of premourning.

Now came the hard part (Mark was starting to feel guilty). Relentlessly, he plodded onward:

Instead of racing home night after night to prepare dinner, I can arrange to meet a few friends after work for a few laughs one night a week. I can prearrange for the day-care person to stay with Dan a

*few extra hours on a specific night, and on that night I can bring home
some high-toned take-out, or hell, even a pizza.*

*The obstacles to this would be guilt feelings about having a good time
when I know Dan is frustrated or depressed over his lack of energy and
lackluster life. Another potential problem would be getting someone
(day-care worker, friend or Phyllis as a last resort) to sit with him while
I'm out having a good time. Would they understand why I'm at dinner
instead of at Dan's side? Would they think I lacked compassion and cast
accusing glances at me when I came home? So what!*

*To get over these obstacles I must realize that I'm suffering from an
opportunistic infection of the spirit, and to beat the infection I must
put guilt aside. I must put aside embarrassment over wanting to go
out. I give so much to Dan already, and a part of me needs to have
my own needs met, to enjoy life without worrying about Dan's
AIDS. I can give more to Dan if and when I'm invigorated and up.
I feel less resentful and more loving and compassionate. I feel ener-
gized, refreshed and renewed and am eager to try to bring my positive
attitude home and into Dan's life. And that can only help him, too,
in the long run.*

*I'm sure that a sensitive caregiver — professional, friend or family
member — can see that I am not ignoring Dan by wanting to have
these physical or mental stretches. If I'm overwhelmed by feelings of
embarassment or guilt because I choose to go out a couple of nights a
week, I'll have a frank discussion about it. I need these outings to
extend the lease on my sanity.*

FORGIVE AND HEAL

"What could you want that forgiveness cannot give? Do
you want peace? Forgiveness offers it. Do you want happiness, a quiet mind, certainty of purpose and a sense of worth
and beauty that transcends the world? . . . All this forgiveness offers you and more." (*A Course in Miracles*) As author
Marianne Williamson so eloquently points out, a heart of
forgiveness is a healing and freeing gift. Life doesn't have to
be so hard. What makes it hard is not the fact of chronic

illness — or the fact of anything else, for that matter — but judgments about and responses to the facts. Harboring resentment and unforgiveness only add to the heaviness in life.

Chronic illness, in itself, has no meaning beyond certain medical facts. And in many cases the facts about a chronic illness are straightforward, even if people don't understand their causes or their ultimate consequences. Cancer means that abnormal cells in the body grow unchecked. Muscular dystrophy means that muscle cells become weak and swollen and cause progressive weakness of the muscles. Diabetes means that the body is unable to naturally regulate the level of sugar in the blood. Is chronic illness tragic? Does it cause bitterness and anxiety? Is it an excuse to give up, to grieve, to die? Not necessarily. Thoughts about tragedy, bitterness, anxiety and death are all judgments about or responses to the facts. Some people die from cancer; others go blind from diabetes. Those are facts. Caregivers project such outcomes for their loved ones based on their judgment and interpretation of the possibilities.

Have you ever noticed that people "wear" chronic illnesses in different ways? Some sink into despair and isolation, projecting the worst possible outcome. Others find that their spiritual lives deepen, that their attachment to money, power and fame fades. Go to a meeting of Alcoholics Anonymous and you're likely to hear recovering alcoholics who say they're thankful for the fact that they became addicted to alcohol. Why? Because alcoholism forced them into a program of recovery, and recovery transformed their lives.

Stephen Levine, in his book *Who Dies?*, quotes Eastern philosophy when he says that people are already dead. By that he means whether or not a person is sick, he or she will die — someday. In fact, each of us is dying each moment. Every thought, feeling and sensation that makes up a person's sense of self is impermanent. They last only a few seconds, a few minutes, a few hours, a few decades. They all pass — in fact, they are passing right now, even as people become aware of them. In that light, savor each passing moment since that's all you truly have.

None of this is to justify or explain chronic illness, or to say that chronic illness is a test of "character." Judgments about any situation determine the way you feel about that situation. And your judgments are not part of the situation — they're part of you.

As a caregiver you're bound to experience anger, bitterness or a host of related emotions. You might get angry at the PWCI for being so demanding and so needy. You may get angry with yourself for losing your temper for not being a perfect caregiver. You can get angry with doctors for not understanding, or angry at the government for not funding research that brings an end to chronic illness.

All this can be a little easier to deal with if you remember that your anger usually comes from judgment. Caregivers usually have highly developed pictures in their minds — pictures about what they want other people to say and do, pictures about how other people must behave to satisfy them. And when people fail to live up to these pictures, resenting them simply for being imperfect is often a natural response.

To let go of anger, you can first learn to be aware of your judging. With awareness comes perspective on judgment. And when you get that perspective, you get a taste of forgiveness.

What happens when you stop judging yourself and others for not being perfect? Look back on your own experience of forgiving someone else. Chances are you felt a tremendous burden being lifted. You found out that carrying a grudge takes a lot of energy. Forgiveness means you free up that energy, that you're able to turn your attention to other matters, that you can go on. Chances are you could laugh again, that your muscles lost some tension and you could breathe easier. These are all benefits of forgiveness — benefits that can help you every day you care for someone with chronic illness.

Forgiveness doesn't mean you become a doormat. It doesn't mean that you become passive and let people walk all over you. No. You're still free to act, to point out injustice, to be assertive and to express your feelings. You can do all these things without the extra baggage of resentment. You can be lighter, free and more effective in everything you do. You allow others to be as human and imperfect as you are.

Remember that avoiding people with whom you're angry is not the same as forgiving them. What's more, these people are taking up space in your brain rent free.

In their book *You Can't Afford the Luxury of a Negative Thought,* John-Roger and Peter McWilliams suggest that people wait five years before judging anyone or anything. In addition, they say people can declare periods of general amnesty during the day — times when they promise to immediately forgive any wrongs and let go of resentments. The idea is to start with a few minutes each day and keep expanding the time until "zones" of forgiveness occupy much of people's lives.

You are human. You make mistakes and so do other people. It is essential for you to accept your humanness and the fallibility of others. When you err, you can forgive yourself; in fact, you must if you are to stay sane! When the doctor, a friend or the PWCI err, you can be just as ready to forgive them.

Sometimes you will be hurt by others, even if they mean no harm. They may have no idea that you are hurt or angry, or why you feel that way. Or perhaps they did mean harm. Their motivation is less important than your response to their behavior.

Don't forgive others because it is a "nice" thing to do. Forgive *them* in order to heal *yourself,* to open up your world, your heart. The ability to forgive yourself and others enhances your ability to connect with other people.

Application 28: Working With Feelings

Declare "amnesty zones" — periods of time when you promise yourself to forgive anyone you're angry with and let go of resentments. Just start with a short time period — fifteen minutes or a half hour. Then gradually lengthen that period up to 24 hours. Note the results: Do you find yourself less agitated, irritable or tired during your amnesty periods? After working with this exercise for a while, consider increasing your amnesty zones to one week or even one month.

Application 29: Working With Feelings

Are you hiding anger from yourself? Read through the following list and consider whether any of the items describe current situations in your life. Do they point to an unexpressed anger that you feel? If they do, first become aware of them and write them down.

- Procrastination in completing a task
- Habitual lateness
- A preference for sadistic or ironic humor
- Sarcasm, cycnicism or flippancy in conversation
- Frequent sighing
- Over-politeness, constant cheerfulness or an attitude of "grin and bear it"
- Smiling while hurting
- Frequent disturbing or frightening dreams
- An overcontrolled monotone speaking voice
- Difficulty in getting to sleep or sleeping through the night
- Boredom, apathy, loss of interest in things about which you are usually enthusiastic
- Getting tired more easily than usual
- Excessive irritability over trifles
- Getting drowsy at inappropriate times
- Chronically sore or stiff neck or shoulder muscles; stomach ulcers
- Facial tics, habitual fist clenching or spasmodic foot movements

Application 30: Taking Action

Now create a plan for identifying these behaviors, noting them and letting them go.

In this book you'll find the phrase "letting go" used more than once. Letting go is a skill you'll be asked to use countless times — letting go of the familiar routine, of your sadness, your anger, your resentments, your expectations.

Those two words — *letting go* — roll easily off the lips. Yet putting them into practice is not nearly so easy. Fortunately there is one meditation technique that you can use to increase your skill in letting go. What's more, it's a skill you can practice with the PWCI: co-meditation.

Don't let the word "meditation" scare you. There's nothing dogmatic or religious about this technique. It can easily become part of any spiritual practice you have now. On the other hand, you do not have to consider yourself a spiritual person in order to use it.

One by-product of any meditation technique, including co-meditation, is a state of serenity and calm — a state you can access even in the most stressful life circumstances. Co-meditation uses awareness of the breath as a means to promote this calming state. More specifically, you will become aware of both your breathing and the breathing of the person for whom you care.

There is an important link between your breathing and your mental and emotional states. When you're agitated, restless or angry, your breathing will usually be short and clipped. On the other hand, when you're relaxed, confident and open to the world, your breathing will usually slow down and expand. If it's true that emotions influence breathing patterns, then you can use the process in reverse: You can pay attention to your breathing patterns, aiming to influence your emotional state.

Co-meditation is based on sharing a breathing pattern with the person for whom you care. After finding a quiet, dimly-lit place where the two of you can be alone, you will function as the guide for the co-meditation session and offer some introductory suggestions for relaxing. Then you will concentrate on the breathing pattern of your PWCI. The result for most people is a marked decrease in respiration, a slowing of mental activity, profound relaxation and often a spiritual connection.

The co-meditation technique works simply. These instructions are adapted from *Letting Go: A Holistic and Meditative Approach to Dying:*

1. Ask your PWCI to lie on the floor or a firm bed, with hands free and resting next to the thighs, palms up. This person's eyes should be shut.

2. Let any conversation come to a close naturally. After a few moments of silence, slowly offer a series of relaxation suggestions. Simply start with "relax the toes . . . continuing to the ankles . . . knees . . . hips . . . pelvic area . . . stomach . . . chest . . . shoulders . . ." Continue, naming areas of the body up to the scalp and forehead. Then ask your PWCI to become aware of the whole body and let it relax.

3. After the relaxation, observe the PWCI's breathing. If it is still rapid, then proceed with more relaxation suggestions. Here is what you can say:

   > We are now going to share an ancient method of calming the mind and body. There is nothing to fear. I am going to remain beside you. You will not be alone.
   >
   > Now then, while your eyes remain closed, I want you to pay close attention to the sound of my voice. There is nothing else for you to do except listen carefully to my voice and follow your own breathing.
   >
   > We are now going to begin, together, the great sound of "letting go," the word "ah" sounded out and strung out like this: aaaaaaaaaahhhhhhhhhhhh. With each out-breath or exhalation, I will sound aaaaaaahhhhhhh.
   >
   > Please, now think of nothing but the sound of letting go. Thinking is not needed. Just hear the ah and notice your breathing. Just the ah and your own breathing. Allow everything else to fall away from your mind.

4. Now focus your attention on the the PWCI's lower chest area and observe the person's breathing rate. Be sure to begin sounding the aaaaahhhhhh just as your PWCI's exhalation begins. Match your PWCI's breathing rate. It's as if you're doing a very slow dance with your PWCI, with the only movement taking place in your chests and diaphragms.

5. If your PWCI is still breathing rapidly, try counting breaths. You can say:

> Now we will start to count your out-breaths, going from one to ten and repeating the series. I will do the counting for you. All you need to do is follow the numbers with your mind and breathing. Thinking is not necessary. Just counting and breathing . . . counting and breathing.
>
> You may find it helps to visualize a large white number — one through ten — appearing over your head as I count. This might help you focus on your breath.

As you say these words, notice the rise and fall of your PWCI's chest. Synchronize your counting with the other person's breathing, so that they become one. As his or her breathing slows, resume sounding ah with each exhalation.

6. If your PWCI falls asleep, that's fine. Simply continue to breathe and sound ah with each exhalation.
7. Continue breathing for a comfortable length of time. Twenty to thirty minutes is a good length of time for this exercise.

Co-meditation is an age-old technique that fosters intimacy with little effort. Caregivers can enhance their relationships with PWCIs through this and other techniques found in this chapter, while watching for co-dependent behaviors.

5 JOURNALING:
Discover What You Already Know

While caring for someone who is a PWCI, you get to learn a lot, not only about the illness but about yourself as well. The problem is that much of what is learned can be forgotten or obscured by the daily demands of caregiving tasks. It's possible to forget what you know, to lose contact with your inner wisdom. Keeping a journal can help you catalogue your new wisdom and remain grounded.

Many people live with a head and heart full of half-formed and half-expressed wishes, feelings and ideas. And often they are not aware of the behavior patterns that create feelings of joy or suffering in their lives. Writing is a way of bringing clarity to thinking and feeling. Keeping a journal shines a light on what's inside you and brings it into sharper focus. Writing also reveals patterns in your life — healing patterns as well as patterns you can choose to change. Through journaling, as novelist Anais Nin pointed out, you "taste life twice" — first in the experience, then in savoring or coming to terms with that experience.

ROSE, ELSIE AND MICHAEL

Rose's shrink, handsome Dr. Wilburforce, was from Kentucky and had a rolling drawl of humor and insight dry as country dust. She had been going to him weekly for the past eight months, her initial visits instigated by guilt and anxiety about her parents and her resentment toward Paul and his "entitled" wife.

Dr. Wilburforce gave Rose a written homework assignment. She was to write about the impact illness had on her as a child and its impact on her life today. Rose couldn't wait to get back to the Park Avenue apartment to begin the assignment.

Rose could not recall anything about her maternal relatives. But she recalled her paternal grandfather's painful bout with cancer. Back then, and still in some unenlightened circles today, the "c - word" was never uttered. If anything, the word was ventriloquized. The mouth would move forming the word while the larynx remained vibrationless. At age seven she was shielded from the horrors of pain and sickness, but she recalled the doctor's frequent visits that winter, her grandfather's screams in the night and an eavesdropped conversation about what to tell the business partner, family, friends and neighbors. Such was the attendant ignorance and shame surrounding cancer. Rose remembered asking her father if Grandpa did anything wrong and being told, "Mind your own business." She wondered about all the whispers and mystery.

She recalled the funeral and mourning and the torrents of food and company. She recalled her parents' and grandmother's grief. But she did not quite understand it. All she was told was that her grandfather would no longer be around, that he was gone. Because her parents had been so protective, there was no need for an explanation about suffering and death. They meant well, she was sure.

When Rose came down with measles and had a fever, she was coddled and her parents doted on her. The doctor was summoned at once, and her grandmother, mother and father seemed ever-present at her bedside, applying lotions, cold packs, spooning in liquids, singing. "Even Paul was press-ganged into battle to fight my fever. Grudgingly he too changed compresses," she wrote in her notebook. "Maybe the schmuck thinks his responsibility to his family ended at age nine." Her resentment toward her brother was plain.

And she reflected that nothing had changed over the decades. Her father was still protective and secretive, reluctant to divulge the nature or the extent of her mother's illness — forever minimizing its gravity in front of people but performing Herculean feats in ministering and caring.

"How many times," she wondered and wrote, "did Ma have episodes of mental lapse? How often did she wander from the apartment, or worse, from the building and onto the street? I know damned well that he's not telling us the half of it." Rose remembered an oxymoron from some English lit class, *the child is father to the man*, and wrote:

How this really applies. He was protecting us from the pain of sickness and hurting back then as he is now. He doesn't want us to know. I wish I didn't know anything about it, but I do. I know too much. I can no longer deny what is happening to her or to him. And I cannot deny my responsibility. I am in for a very rough time and probably an unpleasant one, especially with Pa and Paul and that witch he's married to.

Rose was diligent in following Dr. Wilburforce's directive about journaling. "Jot down notes about any relationship

that's troubling you," he instructed. Rose composed a litany.
High on the list was Paul and his ill-natured bride.

Rose continued writing:

*Paul and that woman have plenty of room and plenty of money and
they have that live-in maid who could help. But they will have none
of this. I can't have Pa and Ma stay with us. Pa never got along with
John and our apartment is too small. We'd have to convert the den into
a bedroom and they'd have to share a bathroom with Brandon. Three
people sharing a Park Avenue bathroom. It's like something out of
Tobacco Road. Paul has to take the bull by the horns and insist that
either Pa and Ma go into a nursing home or go live with him. It is
evident to everyone that Pa and Ma can no longer be by themselves.*

Rose began to record her own response to the situation:

*I feel helpless, frustrated and resentful. Frustrated that Pa is so
proud and stubborn, helpless because I am in New York and they are
in Florida and resentful that Paul is doing the bare minimum. His wife
is no help, and for her I feel contempt. Lisa and Dr. Wilburforce both
think the entire family should have a face-to-face discussion after Paul
and I come to some agreement on this matter. Fat chance! But Lisa and
Dr. Wilburforce think it's worth another try.*

Rose continued to follow Dr. Wilburforce's instructions
and made a list, dividing the components of the situation
into me, him and us.

Me	Him	Us
1. *Far away*	*Far away*	*Distance is a problem*
2. *Have some money to spend*	*Has lots of money. Can pay for nursing if we're all willing to part with the money*	*Money no big problem*
3. *Willing to help — he doesn't believe me*	*Says he's willing but I don't believe him*	*No trust* *Polarized*

| 4. Not as much time as needed. Hard to get away from N.Y. | Can't leave job. Thinks I am lazy and can go to Florida whenever I want | Neither has or is willing to make such a time commitment |

As Rose was making the list there was no need to check it twice. The options were limited and crystal clear. She and Paul would have to take time and meet in Florida very soon. They would jointly have to find a safe living situation or supervised living setting where their folks wouldn't feel out of place. It would need to be near the water and comfortable and they would need to establish a joint son/daughter front to fight off their parents' certain resistance to the plan.

Next, she mapped out some ideas on handling the cost. They would, she wrote, split it three ways. Pa, her and Paul. They would have to sit down, just she and Paul, and talk about this and try to get rid of the resentments that had been fermenting for so long. Yes, they must have a talk. Perhaps they could find someone as understanding and helpful as Dr. Wilburforce to help them talk through some of the issues. She jotted herself a note to ask Dr. Wilburforce if he knew a good shrink in Florida (but she would use the term psychiatrist since Dr. Wilburforce had asked her not to refer to him as a shrink because it made him sound small).

She wondered if her stubborn father would go for the idea of giving up his place. After all, they were comfortable there, had friends there and her mother would have trouble making such a big change. She felt her resolve slipping a bit and wrote out an alternative. Perhaps they'd investigate Paul's last idea — a day-care center for Alzheimer's disease sufferers, staffed by caring professionals and federally subsidized. She knew that her mother could no longer be left in the hands of untrained "baby-sitters," cook/cleaners who had been hired and fired so many times in the past.

So she'd offer her father a choice. He'd like that much better than being told what to do. Proud of herself, she shut her expensive journal and grabbed her purse, late for her third manicure appointment that month.

JOURNALING PROMOTES AWARENESS

Through journaling Rose was able to sort through complex emotions and conflicting feelings. There's some evidence that journaling has healing effects that penetrate the body as well as the mind. James Pennebaker, a psychology professor at Southern Methodist University in Dallas, has studied the effects of "confessional writing" on health. He conducted research in which a group of student volunteers kept a journal for four days, writing 15 minutes each day. These people wrote about either superficial or traumatic experiences. Those who wrote about traumas, in turn, were further divided into three groups: those who (1) just wrote about their emotional reactions to the traumatic events, (2) just described the facts of those events and (3) wrote about both the facts and emotions.

As Pennebaker tells it, many of the latter group wrote stories that depicted profound human tragedies — stories of sexual abuse, reactions to parents' divorces, alcoholism and suicide attempts. Several people who took part in the study cried as they wrote. Others reported repeated dreams about the subjects of their writing.

Did writing help people work through their feelings? Well, not at first. It was common for the students to report they felt worse immediately after writing, not better. Four months later, however, the same group completed questionnaires about their emotional health. Pennebaker found that emotional health had improved — a result he attributes to the writing these students did.

Pennebaker also wanted to know if confessional writing had any effect on physical health as well. He asked the student health center to keep records of how many times each student had visited the center. Before the experiment took place, the students visited the health center at nearly the same rate. But six months after the experiment those who wrote about traumatic events and their emotional reactions visited the health center only half as often as before the experiment.

Pennebaker didn't stop there. He teamed up with an immunologist and clinical psychologist to see if this type of writing could actually improve resistance to disease. This time the researchers drew blood samples from each of the students who kept journals — one day before they started writing, one day after the last writing session and another sample six weeks later. Each time their blood was analyzed to measure T-lymphocytes, natural "killer cells" that fight off disease. The results: People who wrote about their emotions and traumatic experiences showed a heightened immune response.

This is not to say that keeping a journal will keep you free of disease or discomfort. Writing is not a cure-all. However, writing about your deepest feelings — even those you'd hesitate to share with a close friend — helps you stand back from events. You can see things with more detachment, more perspective. You can see how the events of your life add up in a way that makes sense. And from that new viewpoint, you can choose new ways to act.

One of the students who took part in Pennebaker's study put it this way: "Although I have not talked with anyone about what I wrote, I was finally able to deal with it and work through the pain instead of trying to block it out. Now it doesn't hurt to think about it."

Writing a journal is a hero's journey down the most exciting path anyone can take into his or her interior self. There's no predicting where that path will lead you or what discoveries you'll make. For example, writer Sylvia Fraser remembered that she'd been an incest victim only after writing five novels and noticing that her books contained a lot of sexual violence.

On the other hand, discoveries can be lighthearted and liberating as well. Reflecting on how you've survived tough times in the past can reveal hidden reserves of strength. Viewing your life over the decades, you can realize just how competent and resilient you really are.

HOW TO WRITE A JOURNAL

There is no "correct" way to journal. Call it what you will — journal, notebook, day book, diary. All these terms are interchangeable. Your entries can be a detailed account of the day's events, two lines of poetry, a single paragraph, one sentence, some random doodling, a prayer or a promise that you'll soon take a break from caregiving responsibilities. The only essential is to make contact with yourself regularly through writing.

Some useful guidelines for beginning are:

- Write at a place and time where you're free from interruptions.
- Don't worry about quality or quantity. No one needs to see what you write unless you choose to reveal it. You're free to write whatever comes into your mind.
- Write when you feel the desire. There's no requirement to write every day. But do write when you find yourself dwelling on some event or thought too much of the time.
- Use your journal for your most intimate thoughts. Your journal won't judge you. It's completely open-minded and accepting. And it's available 24 hours each day — free.
- Do timed writing. Set a stopwatch for, say, ten minutes. Write for that whole period without letting your hand leave the paper. Don't stop to edit, cross out or

change grammar, spelling or punctuation. Stick to
your "first thoughts."

- If you can't think of anything to write, then write
  about that. Write anything to begin with. The mere
  act of moving pen across paper or finger over the
  keyboard will prime your mental pump.
- Encourage the PWCI to keep a journal as well. Set
  aside times where you write together. (Be careful not
  to base what you write on what the other person
  writes.)
- Don't worry if you feel sad immediately after writing.
  According to Pennebaker, these feelings usually go
  away in anywhere from an hour to a couple of days.
  If strong negative feelings persist longer than this,
  then talk to someone — a close friend, family member
  or counselor.
- If you want, include more than words. Make charts,
  diagrams, cartoons and drawings.
- Remember that journals can be in formats other than
  the traditional diary kept under lock and key. Scraps
  of paper, index cards, backs of envelopes — all are
  appropriate for journal entries. You may even wish to
  keep an electronic journal: Record your ideas on a
  cassette tape or type them into a personal computer.

WHAT TO WRITE ABOUT

Just as there are no set rules for how to write a journal,
there are no rules for what to write. Here are a few ideas
to get you started.

- Clip articles from newspapers and magazines and paste
  them in your journal. Reflect on what you're reading.
- Copy your favorite quotations or extended passages
  from favorite writers. Doing so may prompt some of
  your own reactions to the writer's ideas. Write those
  down, too.

- Choose some "leading sentences" and complete them with the first thoughts that come into your head. (Example: "The most important thing I could say to another caregiver who wants to stay sane is. . .")
- Keep a gratitude list — a list of people, events and things for which you're grateful. Doing this is more than an exercise in superficial "positive thinking." Instead, gratitude lists are based on a simple principle: What you think about expands. If you dwell on what's missing and what's wrong with your life, those conditions become more prominent in your life. But if you set aside brief times to remember what's going well, then this reorients your thinking. And the quality of your thinking — that is, the way you choose to react to events — largely determines the quality of your life.
- Make other lists: lists of goals. Lists of tasks to complete. Lists of things you want or things you miss. Even such mundane items as grocery lists or laundry lists can help you sort out and organize what you were doing during certain periods of your life. It also gives you a sense of accomplishment when you get things done.
- Write a vision of the future. Write about what you want to do, have and be in six months, one year or ten years from now. Be specific: Pick a day and write what you will do each hour of the day. What will you see, taste, touch, smell or hear? Where will you live? What does that place look like? What people will be in your life? What will you do besides caregiving? Or will you even be a primary caregiver anymore?

The things you create vividly in your mind have a greater chance of actually coming to pass in your life. Goals, wishes and aspirations that are vague and half-formed may remain just that. But detailed mental pictures can move you into action — even when you're not aware of those pictures.

- Track your attitudes. As mentioned before, your attitudes about events — and not the events themselves — often determine how you feel. And the daily changes that come with chronic illness can put you on an emotional roller coaster. Therefore, a useful way to write is not only to record the events of your daily life, but your attitudes toward them, much like the students in Pennebaker's study.

  One of the kindest things caregivers can do for themselves is to notice their attitudes. Just seeing the up and down swings in your attitudes can provide a calming perspective. Caregivers often notice that there are breaks even in the bleakest depressions. Bad feelings seldom last forever. They're not solid or permanent. Seeing this over and over again might loosen the grip of negative emotions the next time they come around.

- Write affirmations. If it's true that what people think about all the time comes to pass in their lives, then it pays to think thoughts that heal and empower. To write an effective affirmation note something specific that you want to do, have or be. Then describe yourself as if the change has already taken place:

  "I am a competent caregiver."

  "I take time off for myself every day."

  It also helps to express ideas positively. Instead of saying "I am not fat," say:

  "I am eating carefully every day and am achieving my weight goal."

  Finally, experiment with memorizing your affirmations or posting them in places where you'll see them often. Repeat them when you wake up or just before you go to sleep.

WRITE ABOUT DREAMS

Dreams can be nightly "bulletins" from a person's deepest self. And in some cases, they guide a person to healing actions and attitudes. Psychologist Patricia Garfield studied the dreams of people who were ill or injured. She found that each stage of illness and the return to wellness may be charted in dreams. "Each organ in the body has a voice in a dream," she writes. "In fact, when a person's body becomes disturbed, dreams are often the first to know."

Sometimes, for example, people's dreams provided a warning or predicted an illness or injury. Common images included driving a car fast with no brakes, being warned by a wise figure to slow down or fainting while clinging to a window ledge. In general, Garfield concludes, these dreams indicate that a person is going too fast, nearing the point of exhaustion or confronting danger. These are signs to heed.

Besides offering warnings, dreams can also signal a return to emotional or physical health. People with these kinds of dreams reported dreaming about a beautiful view from a window, driving safely on a hazardous road or planting a garden.

Dreams form a perfect subject for journal writing. First, plan on remembering your dreams. Repeat this intention during the day, especially as you fall asleep. It helps to keep a notepad and pencil or a small tape recorder by your bed. Use these to record your dreams. In order to improve your dream recall Garfield suggests keeping your eyes closed as you write or dictate.

Some people ask questions or make requests to be fufilled in dreams. There is an ancient practice called "dream incubation" that guides people in precisely how to do this. Some keys to dream incubation are keeping a journal of dream requests ("What direction shall I take next? Comfort me."), repeating your request as you fall asleep and imagining that your request will be fulfilled when you wake up. Note that this process may take several tries. Moreover, it's wise to use clear-headed judgment about any "advice" you get from a dream.

INSIGHTS AND INTENTIONS —
HOW TO FOLLOW UP

If you write regularly, your journal will become a well of insights. It's worth plumbing that well from time to time. That means rereading your journals once every few weeks, months or years.

After all, human beings have a habit of forgetting. Sometimes people repeat mistakes merely because they forgot the lesson they learned the last time around. It's not unusual to forget the insights that brought a host of issues into sharp focus. People forget the insights and events that prompted major shifts in their life's direction. They forget the best things that others have told them. Keeping a journal and rereading it makes all those moments available again.

One thing many journal writers notice is that they forget to follow up on their best ideas. Even the grand "ahas!" can get lost in the daily shuffle, especially by tired and over-worked caregivers. Besides offering pleasurable reading, reviewing your journals can resurrect these gems.

It helps to view your journal entries as falling into two basic categories: insights and intentions. Insights are ideas to remember, things to keep in mind. Rereading your journal from time to time will help you keep track of those.

Intentions, however, are something else. These are entries that call for some follow-up, some further action or attention. Examples include to-do lists, questions to ask the doctor, plans for a vacation, phone calls you want to make and any other goal or task you want to complete.

The first step to following up on these intentions is becoming aware of what they are. As you reread your journal, mark them with an A (for action) or an I (for intention). Highlight them, underline them — do anything to make your intentions stand out. You can do this quickly, in just a few minutes. And don't worry about catching all your intentions. Whatever you miss, you can catch the next time around.

Next, use a pocket diary or calendar book and schedule time for your intentions. Caregivers commonly load their schedules with tasks to complete for others — groceries to buy, appointments to keep, people to contact — and forget the tasks that benefit them. Write down "appointments" with yourself to read, meditate, walk, exercise, play or do nothing at all.

Some intentions are grand: "Take charge of my health." "Think about myself for a change." "Connect to other people more often." "Take a two-week vacation." To bring these intentions to bear in your life, translate them into immediate tasks — actions you could take today or within the coming week. For example, the intention to take a vacation can translate into "get a brochure from my travel agent" or "make a list of places I'd like to visit."

Finally, don't feel obligated to follow up on all your intentions. Taking one follow-up action each week or each month is fine. As a caregiver the last thing you want to do is load yourself down with more chores. Rather, choose those intentions that will have the greatest impact on your quality of life. That may mean only one or two out of every ten or twenty intentions.

GET YOUR HAND MOVING

The rest of this chapter offers suggestions and examples of journal entries. Scan through them all and pick one that attracts you. Later you can come back and choose others. Also feel free to ignore these suggestions and to write about what's "up front" for you right now.

Application 31: Learning

Write a "job description" for yourself as a caregiver. Make it sound like the description for a paid job. Include the tasks you complete as well as the skill and knowledge that's required for your "position."

After writing your description, give yourself a pat on the back for taking on and successfully completing such a difficult job. Then look over your list of responsibilities. Are you trying to do too much? Where can you set limits? Are certain tasks beyond your present knowledge or skill level? Where could you use some help?

Create a "job description" for a "helper." See where you can secure some of that help and arrange to get it.

PEARL, RITA AND JACKIE

Over the next months Pearl had many more conversations with Mrs. Goodwell, checking in on Jackie's school attendance, her classroom deportment and her grades. Pearl enjoyed the conversations with Mrs. Goodwell because news of Jackie's spring back was pleasing. During these conversations Pearl always picked up a technique or two to either help her with the caregiving process or to strengthen the bond with her grandchildren. Above all, she learned from Mrs. Goodwell that she must put Rita's illness in perspective and view it within the context of the family.

Pearl learned that she didn't have to be at Rita's hospital bedside eight hours a day. In fact, Rita felt relieved to know that Jackie and Joey were being so well cared for by their grandmother. Instead of having to worry about her children, Rita could concentrate all her energy toward healing herself.

Homework done, tonight's exercise for Pearl and Jackie was to write a job description for caregiving. They would write it together. The night was star clear and the old woman gazed out the window, pondering before licking the tip of the pencil and writing.

HELP WANTED: CAREGIVER. Patient, loving caregiver wanted for young woman with Hodgkin's disease. Must be willing to work long hours and meet emergencies.

"Must have a driver's license," offered Jackie. For her sixteenth birthday, Rita and Pearl arranged for her to go to driving school and have private lessons. Jackie could now drive until sunset.

"Must like children ages 15 and 10. Must have a strong stomach. Must be willing to cook, clean, do laundry for two adults and two children. Must be willing to sit with an eight-year-old boy. Must have counseling skills and be willing to listen to loud music on the radio."

Pearl and Jackie laughed at this last requirement. What Pearl also wanted to add was "must be able to whistle while running past the graveyard, must be able to go from raft to tempest, from peak to valley." And it was these last, unwritten job qualifications that Pearl knew she possessed in abundance. She never permitted death to sniff around and depression didn't dare darken her door. In this house the cup was always half full, at least if Pearl had anything to say.

Pearl and Jackie looked over the job description. Pearl said she was relieved that Jackie had received her driver's license. It was a big help having Jackie drive to the market or other stores. Such errands always taxed Pearl and cut into hospital time. Pearl further commented that some months ago she had been negligent in the child care department, but that was past now thanks to Mrs. Goodwell's alert, Pearl's willingness to reset priorities and Jackie's positive response to the situation.

Pearl also knew she was good at putting on a happy face. In fact, she could act as if it were New Year's Eve squared in her heart. Even though her counseling skills were rudimentary and limited, she could easily give pep talks to Rita, Jackie and Joey. There was no end to the various reassurances that sprang to her lips to ward off the spectre of tragedy.

Application 32: Learning

Write a letter to another caregiver. Offer your ideas on how to be a skilled caregiver and stay sane in the process.

As a variation on this exercise, write a letter that focuses on a certain emotion or person. For instance, write a love letter to the person you care for. Or write a love letter to yourself. Write a letter expressing anger, sadness, grief or any other strong emotion you feel.

When you're done with the letter, reread it. Have you gained a new perspective on your feelings? Has the intensity of your feelings changed? Have you learned anything? Consider sharing all or part of your letter with someone else.

Application 33: Learning

Coach yourself. Imagine that you're speaking to another caregiver who's facing the same problem you face right now. What would you say to this person? (This exercise can be even more fun if you do some role-playing and actually involve another person as the person you're coaching.)

Application 34: Learning

Write a letter from the perspective of the PWCI. Enter that person's world. Describe what it feels like to have a chronic illness. Describe that person's daily routine.

After finishing the letter ask if you've learned anything new about the person you care for. Does anything you've learned call for a change in your caregiving approach? Consider reading all or part of this letter to the PWCI.

Application 35: Learning

Write a contract for your job as a caregiver. Imagine you're an outside consultant who's agreed to take on the role of caregiver. Specify your working hours. Determine what you'd charge for your services based on prevailing rates in your area. Spell out what tasks you agree to do. Also list what you will not do — the tasks that you consider beyond your role as a caregiver.

Now look over your contract. Does it spell out more tasks than you're doing now? Less? After doing this exercise, is there anything about your caregiving role that you want to change?

Application 36: Learning

Write a certificate of achievement for yourself as a caregiver. Make it look as official as possible. Print it in fancy script, by hand or, if you have access to one, on a computer.

Application 37: Learning

Make a list of all the tough circumstances you've survived. What tools helped you make it through those times? Can you apply those tools today to your job as caregiver?

Application 38: Learning

Get your assumptions out in the open: What do you assume caregiving means? Complete the sentence "A caregiver should . . . " Write the first things that come to your mind without stopping to edit.

After a day or two come back to what you've written in Applications 31 through 38. Does it express a reasonable view of caregiving — one that helps you take care of yourself as well as the person for whom you care? Are there any changes you'd like to make in your approach to caregiving? List them, then think about how to actually make those changes.

This is a good time to stop and review. Take a rest, put down your book and the work you've done. In the spirit of the next chapter take care of yourself, the most important asset you have as a caregiver. And when you are ready, turn the page and continue.

6 SELF-CARING:
Remember Yourself

How do caregivers stay sane? The standard reply is, "Take care of yourself, too." That's fine advice, but incomplete. On some days taking care of yourself might seem as distant an ideal as trying to leap over a building in a single bound. How do you really implement the idea of self-care in daily life?

CREATE A SANCTUARY

Begin by thinking about places. Think about the spaces you move through — your office, the rooms in your house. Have you ever stopped to think about how you feel about these places? When you enter the rooms where you spend most of your time, do you feel invited, welcome, at home?

Many caregivers find that their physical environments affect their moods and outlook, especially if they spend time in places like doctor's offices, nursing homes or hospitals. There may be physiological reasons for this. Research indicates that elderly people who move to nursing homes — where the environment is often sterile and uninviting — can lose some of their mental functioning. Writers on learning and educational psychology frequently mention the importance of an intellectually stimulating environment.

One way you can care for yourself is to enrich your physical environment. This is a wonderful place to begin self-care because you can take concrete actions that bring definite results.

Try creating a "serenity corner," a place that feels nurturing and affirming to you. This might be a bedroom, a study, a den or a meditation room. If your living space is tight, your serenity corner can be one area within a larger room.

Your aim in creating a serenity corner is to set aside a place to do whatever it is that renews you. That might be meditation, yoga or prayer. It could be listening to music, reading, drawing, painting or sewing. The individual activity is up to you. The point is to experience positive feelings regularly in a specific place. If the association between place and positive feeling is strong enough, you might be able to experience the feelings merely by entering the room.

The French novelist Marcel Proust knew this. Smelling a certain aroma one day triggered a flood of memories that later became the basis for his epic *Remembrance of Things Past.* What is true for the sense of smell is often true for other sense channels as well.

A local writer uses this technique whenever he feels stuck on a project. Normally he works at a computer. But at certain times he'll head for a local coffee shop that sells rolls in the morning and ice cream in the afternoon. Because he's had so many good ideas there in the past, he's come to associate being in this place with getting "unstuck." Merely entering this shop puts him in a different psychological state — one that opens up creative possibilities.

You can use a similar strategy. Create a place where you feel recharged and renewed. Consider the following suggestions:

- Play pleasant music in your serenity corner. If you're not sure what to play, begin with pieces by the Baroque masters, such as Vivaldi, Corelli and Bach. There's some evidence that Baroque music played at medium tempos can have a relaxing effect and actually improve readiness for learning.
- Make use of natural light. Many people respond favorably to sunlight streaming through a window. If you don't have a room that gets sunlight, try to get light from several different lamps placed around the room. Getting most of your light from one source can sometimes cause you to feel like you're being interrogated or that you're under a spotlight.
- Surround yourself with pleasing fixtures. Consider paintings or posters with pastel colors or scenes of nature.
- Send yourself positive messages. Post index cards on the wall with affirmations such as, *"I am a competent and compassionate caregiver"* or *"I turn every problem into a chance to gain new skills."*
- Fill the room with pleasant aromas. The use of scents to alter moods is an ancient practice. It's also simple to implement. Some suggested aromas for relaxing include rose, lavender, orange and chamomile.

CAREGIVING AND CHRONIC ILLNESS TEACH YOU WHO YOU ARE

The following came from a caregiver's journal:

My father died of amyotrophic lateral sclerosis — Lou Gehrig's disease. I remember sitting in the car after the funeral, after everyone that knew him had left, after everything that could be said had been said. Then a thought came to me. I'm not a religious person, but this thought had the character of a revelation. In essence, it was this: You too will die. Now how will you live?

Caregiving is a spiritual teacher. What you learn depends upon your belief system and religious upbringing. It also depends on your capacity to change — to respond, to grow. There is much to learn.

The history of religion is the history of human attempts to learn from suffering. The book of Job, for example, contains some of the most inspired poetry in the Bible, all of it an attempt to answer one question: Why does God allow good people to suffer? That same question preoccupied the Buddha, who made the stark observation that the unenlightened life is "dukkha." This is a word that means being in a state of chronic dissatisfaction, often translated simply as "suffering."

When you care for someone with a chronic illness, observations about the universality of suffering cease to be matters of abstract speculation. Instead, they strike to the marrow of emotional life.

Is there a meaning in suffering? The philosopher Nietzche said: "Man can live with any *how* as long as he has a *why*." That is, if people can see some pattern, some order, some larger perspective in which the fact of suffering makes sense — then many can live more gracefully and stay sane with chronic illness. This is not to say that suffering has any one, universal meaning. Each person grapples with this question of meaning in his or her own way. And each person will integrate his or her own answer to this question into his or her own life. With this in mind, it may be useful to view suffering as a spiritual teacher. Your life with the PWCI is your classroom.

Many caregivers grew up with the ideas that "Suffering makes a stronger person," "Suffering brings people together" or "Suffering builds moral character." Many people hold these ideas to be accurate and powerful. For others they are lifeless, cynical abstractions, phrases that spill too easily from the lips of the able-bodied and the able-minded. Suffering as teacher takes you directly to the core of spirituality. Suffering can teach you about who you are, about the meaning of life.

This book uses "people with" language — that is, people with a chronic illness. Various chapters discuss people with diabetes, people with cancer, people with arthritis or muscular dystrophy. This language is consciously chosen. It underscores that these people are more than an illness. They are, first of all, people.

Another way of saying this is that people are more than their bodies. This is something many people can grasp quite readily. In reality, no aspect of the physical being totally defines who a person is. Some people with diabetes, for example, experience a loss of sensation in their feet. When their diabetes goes uncared for, this can lead to loss of circulation and infection. In some cases the affected foot is amputated. Yet, if people lose a foot to diabetes, a breast to cancer or their strength to muscular dystrophy, have they lost themselves? A person is more than a disease. People are more than their bodies.

The next step may not be so easy to agree with. Even people who do not identify themselves with their bodies may identify with their minds. To say that people are more than their thoughts or feelings is to push personal identity to a new boundary. In other words, are humans truly defined by that passing feeling of jealousy, anger, fear or dread? By that thought of self-pity, that fantasy of revenge, that memory of what's lost to chronic illness?

Many spiritual traditions speak of another part of people called the "witness" or the "observer." It's the place in a person that is aware of being aware. It's the part of a person that can watch emotions and thoughts rise and pass away like waves. From a larger perspective, a wave is a ripple on the surface of a deeper body of water. In a similar way the perturbations of the mind are ripples on the surface of a more quiet, a more interior part of human nature.

In his book *Meditation: An Eight-Point Program*, Eknath Easwaran describes the freedom that comes when a person ceases to identify with the mind and body:

> When you know you are not the body, you find it inaccurate to say, "I'm not feeling well." Your body may be indisposed, but you are always feeling well. Now, in the second stage of meditation, you discover it equally inaccurate to say, "I am angry." The mind is angry. You take full responsibility for your mental states as well as for your behavior.

When you look inside with full attention and full acceptance, you see that nothing about you lasts forever. About every seven years the cells in your body totally regenerate. Moreover, the thoughts and feelings you experienced yesterday have given way to the thoughts and feelings you experience today. You are literally being reborn each day, each hour, each minute.

If chronic illness means anything, it means seeing these things again and again. If you let it, chronic illness can take you to a place where you see a reality beyond your mind and your body. That place has many names: spirit, God, essence, self. Living with chronic illness can enlarge your identity and bring you face-to-face with some larger aspect of yourself, something that transcends the physical, emotional and mental toll of caring for someone with a chronic illness.

It makes your existence meaningful. It makes your life mean more than just suffering. And it converts suffering into an opportunity for you to make contact with your soul. Many caregivers say, in fact, that their spiritual lives began in earnest only after they started dealing with chronic illness on a day-to-day basis. It's from this sense of spirituality that you may be able to cultivate the central skill of caregiving, staying present to the process.

CREATE AN INNER SANCTUARY

Creating an environment that renews and relaxes you is a powerful tool for caregivers. Even more powerful is having a sense of inner peace — a place inside yourself where you can go for serenity. This is an important element to developing spirituality.

There are many ways of creating such a place. For some people it means simply taking a long, hot bath. For others, it means prayer, systematic relaxation, meditation, yoga, visualization and much more. Most of these practices are not tied to a specific doctrine or religious belief. Rather, using them can deepen or extend whatever spiritual orientation you already have. Or these techniques can simply be ends in themselves.

Today there are a multitude of ways to learn such techniques, including books, tapes, classes and seminars. Try several techniques and then select one for regular practice. Whatever technique you choose, aim to practice it daily, at a regular time. Such regular practice will train our mind and body to enter positive states at certain times. For a powerful example, see the instructions for co-meditation on pages 75-77.

PAMPER YOURSELF

Buddhists learn about *metta* and *karuna*, the practices of loving kindness and compassion. They also learn that these qualities are for themselves as much as for other people. In fact, there is a Buddhist saying, "There is not a person in the world more deserving of love than me."

Some caregivers find it easy to take the opposite attitude. They are merciless, heaping upon themselves the kind of criticism they'd never give another person. As a caregiver you deserve to be treated at least as well as the person you care for. Indeed, no one is more deserving of love than you.

Remembering this — and taking regular time off to pamper yourself — can make you a more effective caregiver.

What does taking care of yourself mean? It means taking care of your physical, mental and spiritual health. It means eating foods that give you energy and exercising regularly. In addition, it means playing and taking some time out for blatant self-indulgence.

For example, consider unplugging the phone and taking a long hot bath. Creative activities that involve close sustained attention can also be greatly healing for caregivers. Examples are meditating, praying, reading, listening to music, writing letters, writing a journal, painting, drawing, knitting, working with wood, gardening or sculpting. The key is to choose activities that work for you and set aside specific times for them.

Application 39: Learning

For the next week, monitor the things you say about yourself (both to yourself and to others). Notice statements that include the word "I." Take a few minutes to jot them down daily. At the end of the week go over the things you said about yourself. Would you say these things about another person? Would you say them to the person you care for?

As a result of doing this exercise, do you want to speak differently about yourself? List some new positive statements you'll say about yourself.

Application 40: Taking Action

List five activities that you enjoy — things that refresh and renew you. Choose easy things that are fun and doable. Then list the last time you did each of these activities. Have you done any of them recently? What prevents you from doing any of them now? What can you do to remove those obstacles?

Schedule time for at least one of these activities in the next week. If it's impossible to do the activities you've listed, think of some new ones. Then schedule time for at least one of those activities in the next week.

Application 41: Taking Action

Write yourself a love letter. (If it helps, imagine that you're writing this letter to someone else in the same situation as you.) Congratulate yourself for taking on the various roles in your life, including being a caregiver. Acknowledge the things you do that no one notices. Thank yourself for the skill and knowledge you bring to caregiving.

Keep this letter and reread it from time to time. Consider making a tape of your letter and playing that tape periodically. (You might want to ask someone else to read your letter into the tape recorder.)

Application 42: Learning

Make a list of your roles other than caregiver — for example, wife, husband, lover, father, mother, brother, sister or worker.

Now draw a "pie chart" that represents the amount of time you give to each role in a typical week.

Next, draw a pie chart that represents how much time you'd ideally like to spend on each role.

Finally, compare the two charts. Are there significant differences? What are some specific things you can do to bring your present chart more in line with your ideal chart?

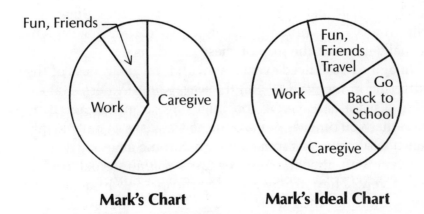

Mark's Chart   **Mark's Ideal Chart**

Application 43: Taking Action

1. List three subjects or activities that interest you — things that have nothing specific to do with caregiving.
2. Next, ask how your day would be different if you were actively pursuing these interests. What would you have that you don't currently have? What would you do that you're not doing now?
3. List any obstacles that currently prevent you from having or doing the things you listed in step two.
4. Finally, list one task you can complete to overcome one of the obstacles you listed in step three. Schedule time for this task within the next week.

USE POSITIVE DENIAL

Everyone has heard about the perils of denial. Everyone has a tendency to turn his or her head away from unpleasant feelings, to ignore, bury, resist and otherwise pretend those feelings don't exist. People are taught that healing can come only when they "get in touch" with those feelings. In order to get past the feelings, you need to allow them full expression. There is merit to this view. Many people are helped by getting past their resistance to negative feelings. Yet continually delving into such feelings can sometimes amplify them. Drowning in pity, anger, sorrow or grief might actually increase the grip of these emotions.

Imagine if you lived every day with total awareness of the suffering in the world — all the war, pain, sickness, starvation, disease and death. You might be so incapacitated by pain that you'd never get around to the tasks of daily living, much less caring for someone with chronic illness.

Every day almost everyone uses *positive* denial to live effectively. They are aware of suffering and injustice. At the same time they don't have to live 24 hours each day with the full reality of all that is wrong with the world. Healthy people take time to listen to music, read, learn, laugh, enjoy relationships and play. Doing so recharges and renews the spirit. Moreoever, it gives you strength to relieve human suffering.

The same idea applies to caregiving. You don't need to live every moment with the full reality of chronic illness in the PWCI. You can remain fully in contact with that reality without dwelling on it or becoming lost in it. Expanding your interests beyond caregiving and talking about other concerns is not denial, but a step toward sanity.

HARNESS THE HEALING POWER OF HUMOR

There is a saying, "The merry heart works like a good doctor." And there's medical truth in this statement. When a person laughs, that person's muscle tension, pulse and posture change. The parts of the body that mobilize in response to stress relax. Laughter also produces endorphins — natural pain killers that are more powerful than injectable morphine. If you pay attention to how you feel when you laugh, you'll notice a subtle healing in the moment.

In addition, laughter provides a form of *positive* denial. It's impossible to be depressed or preoccupied in the moment of laughter. Humor is a sign that you've gained detachment — that you can stand back from your crisis long enough to see it with perspective. With that perspective, you're more apt to see solutions to your problems.

Tears and laughter come from the same place. The problem is that it's too easy to concentrate on the tears and forget the laughter. Many people, especially caregivers, feel the weight of sadness and routine so acutely that they nearly forget how to laugh. At the very least, they often give up the activities that brought them laughter.

You can get past that problem by making time for laughter in your life. Take action to do so. First, search out the things that make you laugh. Watch videos of old funny movies, reruns of "I Love Lucy" or your favorite sitcom or cartoons. Read humorous essays. Do whatever works for you. Use a joy jar, wind up toys, bubbles, a wand or a whoopee cushion. Schedule time for these laughter-producers. Block out a date and time for them, just as you would for a medical appointment or job interview. Making this a regular practice will help you harness the healing power of humor.

Application 44: Taking Action

Experience the healing effects of laughter in a dramatic way. Stand in front of a mirror and laugh as hard as you can for one minute. If you need to, force a belly laugh. Thinking about something funny helps.

When you're finished, lie down, close your eyes and relax. Become quiet and still, both mentally and physically. How do you feel? What changes just took place in your body and mind?

Consider repeating this exercise once a day or several times each week.

Do the same exercise, but instead of laughing, smile. Are the effects any different? How?

Application 45: Learning

Take a humor inventory. Write a list of the five funniest things that have happened to you. Describe them in vivid detail. See them in your mind's eye. Be there once again. Keep a written or tape recorded description of these events and consult them whenever you need a laugh.

MARK AND DAN

Brenda was calling Mark and Dan partly to check on how things had gone at the clinic that day — it was the time for grueling day-long treatments and tests — and partly to vent her anger and frustration. The hospital auxiliary was sponsoring a dance and Brenda had finally got up the nerve to ask a new lab technician if he'd like to accompany her. After all, he was plain-looking and overweight himself — certainly no Adonis or scrubbed Viking. He was a jolly five-by-five type. Brenda had fantasies of a pea-weight romance with high moonbeam content.

But the tech was evasive and noncommittal. When she found out that he later asked a little Thai X-ray tech to the dance, she became depressed. It was not as if Brenda and rejection were strangers, but nonetheless it hurt.

"Let's face it Mark, I'm a 'Dating Game' 4F," Brenda complained. "It sounds like you have Venus envy," Mark said, chuckling at the spontaneous pun. "We are all kind of down around here and I think we could all use a shot of gamma globulin in our jaundiced lives. Come on by tomorrow for a barbeque. We'll grill steaks, make a finicky salad and have some laughs. We'll play a fun game," offered Mark.

Mark went on to explain the nature of the fun fest the three of them would be having the next evening. When he and Dan were down, or even up and in a silly mood, they'd think of silly sounding words, objects, people, places. Invariably, they'd end up laughing. He also told Brenda to recall two or three funny moments in her life and be willing to share them. Brenda hung up and put misery on hold. Fun was on call-waiting and Brenda loved to laugh. That evening she made a list of her funny experiences and made a long list of funny sounding words.

The next evening Dan, Mark and Brenda had a night of abandon and laughter as they went through their lists. The lists of categories and suggestions were limited only by their collective imaginations.

Over cappuccino the three shared humorous experiences: Brenda, at an elegant dinner party hosted by the Director of Nurses, dropped her dangling earring into her soup bowl which splashed hot consomme on the person seated next to her; Brenda getting trapped in a powder room in the middle of a dinner party. The pocket door became hopelessly stuck, and after about 35 minutes it had to be removed. Amidst a roar of laughter, she told about being a weekend guest at the home of her college roommate's parents and having to face the horror of diarrhea and a plugged up, overflowing toilet. "The night before, we had been eating in Little Italy and we didn't roll home until about 4:00 A.M. I should have known that little neck clams and gelato aren't a happy combination," she said, as they all laughed. And in the throes of their uproarious laughter all the pain of the last few months was suspended, if only for a precious moment.

7 CHANGING:

Adapt And Heal

Change does not come easy. Most organisms prefer the certainty and security of a routine. Birds migrate through the same air corridor each year, salmon spawn in the same pattern, pelicans sit on the same part of the sea wall.

So it is with human beings. People often take the same route to work, wear favorite clothing, sleep in a favorite position, develop attachments to others, follow a schedule of personal hygiene and meals. Many vacation in the same place every year with the same people at the same resort. There is an appeal, a comfort level, to a pattern or routine. The Romans said *"Via treta via tuta"* — "The beaten path is the safest one."

CHRONIC ILLNESS IS
A WAKE-UP CALL

When chronic illness enters our lives, people change. They adapt. They leave the beaten path — they have no choice sometimes (getting sick, being physically unable to work, dying). With some things about chronic illness people may sometimes have a choice. Patients and caregivers get to choose which medication to take. They get to choose whether or not to change medications, go to a group, move, change jobs. To maximize the chance of long-term survival change is necessary.

Earlier, we mentioned that the second stage in coping with chronic illness is adapting. Some of the changes caregivers might need to make as part of Stage Two are:

1. Change in the ability to earn money:
   • Inability to work a full schedule.
   • Getting fired because of the need to take care of the PWCI.
2. Change in living environment:
   • Moving to ensure better medical care.
   • Moving to be closer to a support system.
3. Loss of independence:
   • The PWCI may be more dependent as his or her illness progresses.
   • Caregivers may feel obligated and committed to the relationship.
4. Loss of a lover or relationship.
5. Loss of function:
   • Limited energy.
   • Apathy.
   • Narrowing down of social circles depending on who does or doesn't know.
6. Loss of quality of some relationships:
   • People move away in the face of the diagnosis.
   • Caregivers and PWCIs move away from people.

7. Loss of sexual satisfaction and interest in sex:
- The PWCI may be unable to perform sexually or may be uninterested in the possibility.
- The PWCI may undergo marked physical change, perhaps to the point of disfigurement.
- The person with chronic illness may change emotionally. For some this means becoming more guarded or private. Others may seem to gush with feeling constantly in a way that is draining. Some PWCIs get angry and distant. Others become more needy.
- Caregivers may respond by wanting to turn away.

These are changes that may take place in caregivers' lives in response to the diagnosis of chronic illness. As a result of these changes, it is natural to feel uncomfortable. A routine has been disturbed. Certainty has become uncertainty.

Many caregivers assume new roles: friend becomes nurse, husband becomes watchguard, child becomes guardian, counselor becomes cheerleader. Many become lifelines, breadwinners. Caregivers relinquish their roles as lover, equal, independent.

So what is there to do? If caregivers refuse to change in the face of chronic illness, they may become unhappier. If they are unbending, they may break.

Chapter 2 is about accepting, about meeting life on life's terms. When people become skilled at change, they can sometimes accept changes almost immediately as they happen. More commonly, however, change precedes acceptance. There's a lag in time between the fact of the change and the acceptance of it.

An essential conflict of caregivers is holding on versus letting go. To what do they hold on and when do they let go?

In coping with change, one thing to remember is that caregiving for chronic illness does not end life. Rather, it redirects life. It forges new attitudes, new relationships, new priorities. Here one can take a cue from the processes of nature. Nothing in this world is lost. When a leaf, a tree, an animal or a human being dies, its form melts into the earth and becomes the raw material for new living things. Strictly speaking, things don't truly die — they change in form.

If you look at chronic illness and caregiving in your life, you'll see essentially the same process at work. It's true that some things have been lost: perhaps a job, a relationship, money, a sense of security. But if you were open to them, other things have come in their place: a new sense of what's important in life, a new intimacy with the PWCI, an expanded ability to feel with others who suffer as well as more skill at comforting them.

Caregiving is a daily reminder that it's okay to take risks, to leave the safe havens of stability. "Ships in a harbor are safe, but that's not what ships are for." Indeed, sometimes caregivers are so frozen in their routines that only massive chaotic change can free them.

Faced with changes people can create zones of stability — things that remain essentially unchanged in their lives. In addition, they can work skillfully with emotional reactions to change and learn to take change one day at a time.

When dealing with change, you can stop being a passive recipient and start choosing the changes you want. Despite the fact that change can feel difficult and unnatural, you can actually meet change with change.

Application 46: Learning

List the changes that chronic illness and caregiving have brought to your life. How has this chaos helped you re-examine who you are and what you do?

Are there any insights you have now as a result of your experience with caregiving? For example, do you deal with anger differently than you did before chronic illness? Are you more patient? Do you now attach the same importance to making money or career advancement?

Next, ask the PWCI how he or she thinks life has changed. Also ask that person to reflect on how you have changed since becoming a caregiver.

Finally, make a gratitude list. While fully admitting any changes that have brought you pain, describe the changes for which you're actually thankful. Make a point of returning to this list from time to time.

DAN AND MARK

It was 8:00 P.M. on a hot July night. The cicadas were conducting their mad parliament in the trees. Dan was already peacefully asleep and Mark could only hope that Dan would sleep through the night. Mark stared at Dan, now so ravaged by AIDS, frail and emaciated, operating on two cylinders instead of the eight as he had been when they first met. He recalled those days. Both men had beauty and knowledge, skill and taste. They were young enough so that their lives were made of vivid varying moments, each as bright and as separate from the rest as beads upon a string.

How their bodies, health and lives had changed! They once had a lifestyle. Now their lives revolved around clinics, medical tests and medications. It was a constant battle against doom and gloom. They used to have lusty sex. Now, because of lack of energy and loss of libido, there was little sexual contact. Dan was always so fatigued, his collective energy level couldn't charge an electric toothbrush let alone anything else.

Both men had done a lot of playing in their time, thus they figured they might as well be philosophical about the consequences. Fate had punched Dan's ticket. They became more spiritual after the diagnosis and both men, each in his own way, prayed more. What was good about prayer was how it centered the mind. Yes, AIDS had changed their lives and though they were willing to accept those changes, they hated most of them. Dan would feel guilty about the ways in which his illness had shattered Mark's life, sapping him of spirit and spunk. Mark's depression and falling apart only deepened Dan's sense of hurting Mark. Lilting, joyous words and whistles were replaced by despair shaped tones. How could these men not be depressed? All their friends were dying; the death toll was running amok, like Flanders in 1916. The cloud of death shadowed them.

Mark and Dan read over the list of how their lives had changed: diminished income, loss of libido, less grand living space, loss of social life, pain and suffering, depression over impending widowhood. They had to stop living in a state of anticipating grief and loss. They vowed not to become morose or obsessed with death thoughts because that destroys the present.

They began focusing on their enduring love, for it was every bit as actual as the horror that this illness brought on. They made a new list. "As a result of this illness, we spend more time together; we have grown more sensitive to each other's needs and moods; we've become more spiritual, less selfish, more giving." And once again they both expressed an appreciation for their time together. Mark was no longer obsessed with making tons of money. They truly had an enhanced sense of living each moment with a satisfaction for little pleasures — a touch, a fragrance, a special moment.

Application 47: Taking Action

The purpose of this activity is twofold. One is to make small changes and, two, to see how those changes feel. It's important to see where the resistance to change comes up. The idea is that by changing any one thing, you can learn how to change anything.

Write down ten things you do every single day. For example: brush teeth, eat breakfast, shave, shower, drive to work, see a certain person, eat lunch at a certain time and place, go to a specific meeting, open the mail at a certain time, leave work, eat dinner, watch a certain TV show, read the paper, go to bed at a certain time, perform an evening ritual.

After listing these actions pick one that you will change and change it completely. Change the time and the location and the nature of the experience. Change only one thing at first. Make it an easy one at first. Change it, even if it is inconvenient. Take a different route to work. Use the alternate route even though it may be longer. It should be more scenic or enjoyable in some way. Write about the experience.

After you have done this, change something else on the next day, perhaps making it a little more significant.

Reflect on what you've learned from this exercise. Has making small changes taught you any techniques that would be valuable in making larger-scale changes? List those techniques here and describe how you could use them.

Application 48: Learning

Look at ten things about your life that you've wanted to change since illness entered your life. Examples: your employment, the city you live in, the amount of vacation you take, the way in which you prepare your foods, the amount of exercise you get, friendships new and old, how you feel about yourself, your personal habits — smoking, drinking, drugs, biting nails. It's even okay to add "caring for someone with a chronic illness."

Now brainstorm ways that you might make one of these changes. List any possibilities as they come to mind. Work quickly and don't censor. The ideas you list can be large or small. For example:

- Join a self-help group.
- Enter therapy.
- Stop therapy.
- Change therapists.
- Get up 15 minutes earlier to walk.
- Switch to diet soda.
- Call a friend I've been meaning to invite over.

Sometimes people get so locked into behavior patterns that they need a radical shift. One way to shift is to take the behavior you don't like and simply practice its opposite. For example, if you're not demonstrative, be demonstrative. If you're extremely emotional, try to restrain yourself. If you're dependent on others, try to do things alone. If you are a loner, get more involved with people.

From your brainstorm list choose one task that's workable — something you could do today. Make it a priority to carry out that task. After doing so, reflect: Has making this one small change affected your idea of what's possible for you? Are you ready to take on a larger change?

CREATE A "STABILITY ZONE"

PWCIs and their caregivers often find a healing value in structure, ritual, repetition and order. If chronic illness means anything, it means change. It may well feel that nothing stays the same once chronic illness affects the PWCI. Few things are predictable.

That's why establishing routines is so important. When you enter unfamiliar territory, keep something familiar in sight, something that happens each day. This gives you a port in the storm. How do you find such a port or stability zone? Through connecting with what's familiar. This includes:

- Familiar people. Even when you move to a new city or a new job, you can cultivate relationships from the past. Write letters, use the phone, reach out and people will reach back.
- Familiar activities. Establish a daily practice, such as meditating or writing in a journal, to build up your inner reserves. It's best to choose simple activities that you can carry on in many different locations or at different times of the day. And it's equally important to put down the activity when the demands of caregiving take first priority. Make a note to get back to the activity later today, tomorrow or next week.

Include the PWCI in your list of familiar activities. If possible, do things that you both enjoy and do them together. Do things you used to do even if chronic illness makes them harder to do, or modify the activities to fit the illness and the PWCI's capabilities.

- Familiar things. A cherished object, a set of baseball cards, a card or letter, an album or journal or anything else with emotional significance can help you establish some connection with the past. Photographs, home movies and home videos can also serve this purpose.
- Familiar places. Certain places in your life acquire a significance that sets them apart. These are places where a life-changing event took place: a first kiss, a graduation, the birth of a child, a comfortable home. Visit them or visualize them when you take a few moments for yourself.
- Memories. The next chapters deal with the importance of being present in this moment to all that you are experiencing right now. And yet part of what makes up this moment is your memories of the past. In the midst of illness and adversity it may be helpful to conjure up memories of better times — to recall health and well-being, to appreciate what has been. It's fine to visit memories in the form of photos, videos and story telling — these are all important components of healing the pain of loss.

GETTING COMFORTABLE
WITH YOUR FEELINGS

Caregivers typically face a flood of feelings in response to the change introduced by caregiving for a PWCI. Many of those feelings are negative: fear, shock, anger, denial, envy, grief, to name only a few. What's more, when a caregiver cares deeply for a person, he or she can take on the PWCI's pain. When the PWCI suffers, the caregiver can almost feel that suffering as his or her own. On some days their hearts seem to bend, and the caregiver can feel as if he or she is dying a little.

Caregiving puts caregivers face-to-face with their own limitations. Daily they face illness, disability and death. They see the extremes of life as few others do.

But caregiving opens caregivers to joy. Because they see firsthand that life is impermanent, they know that it is sacred. They learn that life is to be lived in this moment, that "this is it." They learn not to take anything for granted. The simple things — being able to walk, talk, care for oneself, work, play — are extraordinarily complex activities that draw on millions of brain cells and hundreds of coordinated muscle movements. They see miracles. They can laugh.

So caregivers experience both positive and negative feelings. As human beings, they have two basic problems with such feelings. They grab on to the pleasurable feelings. They clutch them, hoping that they'll never fade. And they try to resist and push away the negative feelings. Neither strategy works very well. Instead they give more fuel to negative feelings and turn positive feelings from preferences into compulsions.

You can use a more effective strategy in working with feelings, whether positive, negative or neutral. That strategy includes the following steps:

• Name the feeling. Attach a label to the feeling. Don't worry about precision; a quick mental or written note will do. Naming a feeling is one step toward gaining some perspective and detachment. It helps to know you are having feelings — for some people this takes some adjustment. (For more help, refer to Chapter 1.)

• Let yourself feel the feeling. Remember that feelings are neither good nor bad. They just are. Feelings come from a deep part of you that no one fully understands. They don't define you, and you don't have to act on or identify with any feeling. Give full permission for the feeling to arise. Try not to judge or respond at first. Accept what happens.

• Observe the feeling. Touch it, hold it in your hand, taste it, feel it. If you do, you'll see something about its nature: Feelings are made up of thoughts (words and pictures in the mind) and sensations (an ache in the stomach, a tension in your arms, a tightness in your chest). In other words, when you feel strong emotions, you say certain things to yourself, see certain pictures in your mind and register certain changes in your body.

Feelings, like everything else in this world, change. When you investigate any feeling closely, you see that it's not solid or permanent. Rather, feelings are like waves. The thoughts and sensations rise and fall, ebb and flow. They reach a peak and subside. And eventually, their intensity passes away.

You don't have to push back or resist any negative feelings for they are not permanent. They pass. What's more, you don't have to hold on to any pleasant feeling; when it passes away, another pleasant thought or sensation will rise to take its place or memories of the pleasure will return to visit us every once and a while — like a bonus or treat!

In this sense change can be an ally in working with feelings. As meditation teacher Shinzen Young says, "It's not that 'this too will pass.' It's that 'this too is changing right now, in this very moment.' "

Taking these steps will help you absorb and diffuse the impact of a feeling. It often helps to express the feeling — to give it words. You can commit those words to writing, as in a journal, and you can speak those words to a trusted friend, a support group or a counselor.

PEARL, RITA AND JACKIE

Pearl and Rita joined Jackie in the bright family room, filled with Boston ferns, four-foot orange and lemon trees, staghorn ferns and spider plants. Jackie was tending to the plants and bopping to the rap music. Jackie loved tending to the greenery, as much as she loved dancing to the music. Good-naturedly Rita commented, "How can you listen to this awful stuff?" "It lifts my spirits," said Jackie.

The three women decided that they needed a little Christmas in their house and that they would make a list of everything they did that lifted their spirits or gave them that Christmas feeling. Pearl said she loved getting a facial and a manicure. Rita and Jackie joined a chorus of agreement. "Shopping sprees were loads of fun, too," Rita said. The other two agreed. "How about watching a Tina Turner video?" Rita asked, generating very little enthusiasm. "For me, it's listening to a Nat King Cole album. Some of the songs are romantic and melancholy, but they put me in mind of your father and grandfather, and I feel like a schoolgirl — like a carefree senior on her way to the prom," Pearl said.

Jackie said that when they all went to the Japanese steak house and sat on the floor, that was just as much fun as Disneyland for her. Rita and Pearl agreed. Those places were a real treat — where the deft slice and sizzle routines of the smiling Japanese waiters serve up entertainment as well as sustenance.

Rita made a decision. "Okay. This Saturday I'm going to call in a favor." One of her old friends from the TV studio, Lorenzo, was a cosmetologist. She would have him over and she, Jackie and Pearl would have a makeover — facials, make-up, hairdo, nails. Then they would all go out with Joey and eat Japanese.

Application 49: Working With Feelings

List which activities help change your moods for the better. For example: watching TV, taking a nap, going for a walk, listening to music, writing, eating a gourmet meal, calling a friend. Are any of these behaviors a problem — that is, do you indulge in them to the point that they create self-defeating consequences? If not, choose one of these activities and plan to make it a more regular part of your life.

Application 50: Working With Feelings

Look over the feeling vocabulary listed below. Do any of these words describe feelings you're working with now? Practice using these words. The goal is to talk about your feelings with more skill and precision and to become more self-disclosing. Feel free to add to the list. I feel:

- Afraid
- Annoyed
- Lonely
- Miserable
- Nervous
- Panicky
- Depressed
- Enraged
- Irritated
- Mad
- Hurt
- Sad
- Resentful
- Glad
- Peaceful
- Serene
- Calm
- Ashamed
- Guilty

Application 51: Working With Feelings

This is an exercise in recoloring a negative emotion. Emotional states are created, in part, by thoughts, including memories. Take a minute right now to describe a pleasant memory that involves the PWCI. Perhaps you can recall the first time you met or an act of unusual kindness on the part of that person. Describe that memory in your journal or on your tape recorder.

Now, during the next week, make a practice of noting any emotions you feel when you're with the PWCI. Avoid judging the emotions and just give them a simple label: fear, anger, resentment, tenderness, concern. The next time you feel one of these emotions see if you can recall the memory you just described. Did this affect your emotional state in that moment? If your emotional state did change, how do you think the change could affect your actions toward the person? Write down or record your ideas.

ROSE, ELSIE AND MICHAEL

Paul and Rose were having yet another exasperating and hopeless telephone conversation about their parents. Nothing would be resolved. The conversation came to an abrupt halt when Paul said Rose was like some Racine queen, self-absorbed and oblivious to the day-to-day routine. Rose banged the phone. The insulting allusion was not totally lost. Although she didn't quite understand the "racing queen" part, she heard loud and clear the "self-absorbed" slam.

Later that day, she discussed the accusation with her therapist. It was certainly not the first time she'd been labeled selfish. John would frequently say that she was so self-centered she was a city of one! Dr. Wilburforce convinced Rose that perhaps she'd feel better about herself if she were more flexible and giving when dealing with her parents.

"How can I be loving and compassionate when Ma is so burdensome and Pa is so stubborn? Most of the problem would be solved if only they'd move into a nice nursing home in New York," she told the psychiatrist. "I get so angry at them. And I lose my temper every time," Rose said, twisting her hankie.

Dr. Wilburforce suggested that Rose think of a time when her parents did something very special and particularly meaningful for her. Before she spoke to them next, or saw them next, she should reflect on that special memory.

Many things came to Rose's mind, but the thing that really stuck out was the time she was in a car accident while she was a sophomore in college. Her parents had given up an elaborately planned, long overdue vacation to maintain the hospital vigil. They had not been on a vacation since their honeymoon, and here they were, enduring the daily visits from one in the afternoon until eight at night. Both her mother and father agreed they could not possibly enjoy themselves, knowing she was laid up in a hospital, in traction, alone, having to eat all that dull hospital food off trays in that Spartan room.

So they brought her flowers: pert daisies, like emissaries from the sun; lemony spikes of gladiola and magnolia blossoms, as big as tea cups. They cluttered her hospital room with stuffed bunnies and cuddly bears. They supplemented those drab hospital meals with lots of good food, including baskets of out-of-season fruits and table grapes of the palest green.

And from 11:00 P.M. to 7:00 A.M. there was a private duty nurse to fluff her pillow and wipe her brow. Rose's parents were not rich people and this was an extravagance to end all extravagances. But her parents were there for her and with her, as always. Rose's heart was warmed, even though Paul would characterize it as gradations on a refrigerator. Her parents never went on the cruise.

Rose cried at the memory, and she vowed that whenever she called her father, this memory of their selflessness would be in her thoughts. So on an index card she wrote the words "car accident — hospital — no cruise — care, comfort and attention." She would handle the card every time she called her father or spoke to her mother during her mother's lucid moments.

LIVE IN THIS 24 HOURS

If you're familiar with Alcoholics Anonymous, you may know about the importance of certain slogans in that recovery program from addiction: One day at a time. Let go and let God. Keep it simple. Take it easy. Progress not perfection.

All of them apply to the caregiving experience as well. And most of these slogans have a core idea in common: Live in these 24 hours.

Living one day at a time means avoiding playing mental games that can make you crazy. One of the most prominent is "What if . . .?" in all its variations: What if the person I love had never become chronically ill? What if this person dies? What if I have to live the rest of my life like this? What if we run out of money? What if people find out how angry, impatient and lonely I really am? These are just a few of the "what if's" that can seize the caregiver's mind.

It's possible for you to run such worst cases in your mind over and over again so many times that they acquire a kind of artificial reality. The fact is that most of these events will never come to pass. Caregivers often worry for nothing. "Worry," as the saying goes, "is the interest on a debt you may never have to pay." And besides extracting high emotional costs, worry makes life far more complicated.

An alternative is to take caregiving and life as it comes, one day at a time. Your only obligation is to this 24 hours. Your only task is to be as patient, competent and compassionate a caregiver as you can for this 24 hours. And your constant reminder is to **H.A.L.T.** every 24 hours — that is, to never get too **H**ungry, too **A**ngry, too **L**onely, or too **T**ired. If you do these things, you'll lay the best possible foundation for tomorrow.

A verse from the Indian dramatist and poet Kalidasa says it well:

> Look to this day! For it is life, the very life of life. In its brief course lie all the verities and realities of your existence: The bliss of growth, the glory of action. The splendor of beauty. Yesterday is but a dream, and tomorrow is only a vision, but today well lived makes every yesterday a dream of happiness and every tomorrow a vision of hope. Look well, therefore, to this day!

Such is the salutation of the dawn. When you live in the 24 hours, you become the "right size." To worry compulsively about the future is to foster the illusion of your grandiosity. People often act as though they're indispensable, as if no one can take their place as caregivers, as if their actions alone decide the fate of the person for whom they care. You can take a lot of comfort from the fact that you're not that "big," not that important. There's a real freedom in knowing that life can go on without you, especially without constant worrying and frenetic activity.

Application 52: Working With Feelings

Make a list of "what if's." Indulge yourself in the worst cases you can think of — what's the worst thing that may happen? What if he or she dies? What if she goes blind, gets paralyzed, becomes a vegetable.

Application 53: Taking Action

Now, for every "what if" on your list, write next to it the words "but it's not" or "but he or she isn't" or "but it didn't." Follow each with a positive statement about what is real, right now. For example:

What if Christine becomes paralyzed, can't breathe and needs a respirator? But she's not — she can breathe just fine today.

or

What if Ma goes crazy and hurts Pa, God forbid? But she hasn't, and they both love each other today.

Changing is an essential behavior for all caregivers of PWCIs. Illness brings disruption of routines and expectations. This chapter has offered some techniques for the caregiver to explore change and resistance to it. It is through adapting that caregivers can heal.

8 CHOOSING:

Remember That You Are Not A Victim

Viktor Frankl was a psychiatrist in Austria. But in a Nazi concentration camp during World War II, he was prisoner number 119,104. He was sentenced to forced labor, and one of his tasks was to dig a tunnel for an underground water main — alone. For completing that task he got a token worth 12 cigarettes. He avoided starvation by exchanging that token for 12 bowls of soup.

Even though Frankl was separated from his family and stripped of almost every option, he still felt free. He later wrote, "Everything can be taken from a man but one thing: The last of human freedoms — to choose one's attitude in any given set of circumstances, to choose one's own way." Frankl found solace in the beauty of nature, of the sunsets over mountains — something not even the Nazis could take away. He also remembered his friends and family, especially his wife. "I understood," said Frankl, "how a man who has nothing left in this world may still know bliss, be it only for a brief moment, in the contemplation of his beloved." He found meaning in his memories of connection — and for the moment was connected once more.

Some caregivers describe the entry of chronic illness into their lives as the beginning of a new phase in their lives. Some even describe life (or at least the meaningful part of their lives) as beginning for them at that point. There are many different ways to experience illness when one cares for a PWCI. The response to chronic illness that each caregiver has is a function of that caregiver's choices.

CHOOSE YOUR THOUGHTS

Frankl's story talks about choice and change. Even when you cannot change the things that trouble you, you can change your thoughts about them, change your point of view. There are always other ways to view situations in life.

Is the glass half full, or half empty? It's both, and you get to choose how you think of it. If it's half-full, you have half left — a nice thought. If it's half-empty, it's almost gone!

Compare when Stella and Lola were laid off from their jobs. Stella was convinced that this was the worst possible circumstance. "I always louse up the best opportunities," she thought to herself. "And it's not just in my career. It's in my friendships and love relationships, too. There's simply something about me that eventually turns people off and I don't know what it is. Guess I might as well get used to it."

Lola, also fresh out of a job, took a different attitude. "There's a reason for the fact that I got fired. It could have something to do with me. Or it could have been that our company was losing its market share and just had to cut down on staff. After all, several people got laid off besides me. Things like this just happen sometimes. Being without a job temporarily means I'll have time to read that book about career planning I've got at home. I'll have more time to spend with the family and to practice bowling. And I'll have a chance to get a new more exciting job."

Here are two differences in what psychologist Leonard Seligman calls explanatory style. This term merely refers to the way people explain things to themselves. Certain people have a chronically negative style when they explain things. They tend to see the glass as half-empty instead of half-full. They focus on what's going wrong instead of what's going right.

In fact, people with negative styles tend to use three kinds of statements over and over again. These statements make assumptions. They globalize a situation. Some refer to them as "old tapes," as if a tape recorder is playing in their heads:

- "It's my fault." This means taking personal blame for situations that may be entirely beyond your control. In the words of Stella, "There's something about me that turns people off and that's why I got fired."
- "This situation won't change." Beyond assuming blame, negative thinking means losing hope, concluding that things never will get better. Again, Stella expressed this idea with the words, "Guess I might as well get used to it."
- "Things never go well for me. I always louse up the best opportunities," Stella says to herself. "And it's not just in my career. It's in my friendships and love relationships, too."

Contrast these statements with the words of Lola in the following example. Again, there are three key ideas that come across:

- "I am not to blame." Or, in Lola's words, "There's a reason for the fact that I got fired. It could have something to do with me. Or it could have been that our company was losing its market share and just chose to cut down on staff." And even when you make a mistake, you don't have to waste time or energy on blaming yourself. You can simply change your thinking or behavior so the mistake won't happen again.

- "I can do something to change this situation — or my attitude toward it." Lola gets at this idea by saying, "Being without a job temporarily means I'll have time to read that book about career planning I've got at home."
- "Even when things go wrong sometimes, my life can go well overall." Or, as Lola says, "Things like this just happen sometimes."

Human beings are granted a gift shared by no other creature: They can stand back and look at their thoughts. They can ask questions about every thought they notice running through their heads: Is this thought serving me? Does it contribute to my happiness? Or does it focus on the negative? Does this thought open up more possibilities for me? Or is it closing off my options?

This idea really hits home when such questions are applied to thoughts about chronic illness and caregiving. It's easy to tell yourself a lot of negative things. "Things will never get better." "We might as well give up." "We'll never be able to do things we enjoy now." "Christine gets worse whenever I don't spend enough time with her." Again these are the three negative statements identified earlier: "It's my fault." "This situation won't change." "Things never go well for me."

In such moments whose voice is on the tape recorder? Often it's a parent, teacher, sibling — someone from whom you feel disapproval routinely! On the bright side: You don't have to listen to these people. With a little practice you can learn to shut them off — to turn off the tape recorder.

Note that the two explanatory styles represent extremes. Most people are not exclusively negative nor positive in their explanatory styles. Rather, they fall somewhere between the extremes. Many people feel both extremes at once. This happens when they're attempting to think more constructively but still feel the old negative habits of thought "pulling" at them. Psychologists call this cognitive dissonance, a state where thoughts seem to be at war with each other.

Some people, searching for a way to get past negative thinking, try thinking positively. Sometimes that's okay. But sometimes thinking positively feels like pasting on an artificial smile and forging ahead as if nothing is wrong. This is the psychological equivalent of burying your head in the sand.

Instead of thinking positively, you can think effectively. Effective thinking is based on telling the full truth when events trouble you. It means admitting that Rita's cancer has come back, that Christine needs a wheelchair or that, for Mark and Dan, paying the medical bills means giving up a vacation that's already planned.

Effective thinking does not stop there, however. It goes on to do some specific work with negative thoughts. More specifically, it involves taking three steps:

• Detect negative thoughts.
• Dispute negative thoughts.
• Distract yourself from negative thoughts.

As you read, realize that working with negative thoughts can take time. After all, your emotions spring from a primitive part of your brain, one with animal-like instincts. Sometimes doing this work feels like you're training a dog to do new tricks. Trainers know that it takes many attempts before a dog learns the right moves. They work slowly and patiently, offering frequent rewards to the animals and repeating their hand signals again and again. Sometimes rewiring your mental circuits to accept new thoughts can feel just as basic. Revising the tapes requires repetition and hard work. Sometimes you think the recording is erased only to hear it over again in your head.

If you've spent several decades developing negative thought habits, then those habits probably won't change overnight. You may feel like you're trying to train a menagerie of mutts. Even after several weeks of applying these techniques, you might still notice many negative statements in your thinking. Perhaps you'll erase only 1 percent of your negative explanations, and still feel the weight of that remaining 99 percent. Even so, 1 percent is enough to make a difference you can feel. And it is a beginning. It will be important to acknowledge when these changes are occurring and to appreciate the difference — the rewards of your hard work.

DETECT NEGATIVE THOUGHTS

Visualize ineffective thoughts as cassette tapes that start running whenever a certain event occurs. Picture taking the person with chronic illness to a medical appointment and the doctor recommending that this person enter the hospital for some tests. For some people that's like pushing the play button on the tape recorder: "Uh oh — we better prepare for the worst" or "The last time we did this, she ended up staying in the hospital for a whole month" or "Nothing we do will help us get control of this illness."

One of the most powerful ways to deal with such ineffective thoughts is also one of the simplest: Whenever you have a negative thought, just notice it. That's all. You don't have to do anything else for the moment. Just keep track of your negative thoughts.

There are a number of ways to do this. Some people carry around a counter like the ones golfers use to record their strokes during a game. Every time they detect a negative thought, they press the counter. In many cases this mere act of record keeping is enough to decrease the grip of such thoughts.

You don't need any fancy equipment to do the same thing. For instance, you can simply carry along an index card and pen in your pocket and make a tick mark whenever a negative thought crosses your mind.

Another tactic is taking an inventory of negative thoughts once a day or so, simply writing them in your journal. Some people call a friend and speak their thoughts out loud. Either action may be enough to provide a healthy detachment from negative thoughts.

Application 54: Taking Action

Choose a method you can use to signal the occurrence of a negative thought. Some examples: Speak the thought out loud as it occurs to you. Write it down immediately. Bite your lip (not too hard)! Snap a rubber band. Tap a finger. Pinch yourself. Leave the room. Or take a deep breath.

Choose just one method, apply it for one day and tally the number of negative thoughts. If you want, keep tabs for a week. After the week is over, try to assess how it has affected your thinking. Write about these thoughts. Look at trends. Be aware of key times of the day, circumstances or surroundings that trigger them.

DISPUTE NEGATIVE THOUGHTS

One telltale mark of negative thinking is the occurrence of certain key words or phrases such as:

- All
- Every
- Never
- Should
- Have to
- Can't

These words fall into two broad categories: universals and restrictives. People usually have trouble when they use either category.

All, every and *never* are universals. They claim that certain things are always true and that people and situations never change. Some examples:

- Now that Elsie has Alzheimer's disease, we'll *never* be able to walk on the beach the way we used to.
- *Every* time Dan starts to feel worse, he acts the same way.
- *All* doctors are alike. None of them understand how to deal with Rita's Hodgkin's disease and our feelings. They *never* have and they never will!

When you hear the words *all, every* or *never*, let them be an automatic signal to exercise some critical thinking. Whenever you hear a statement using one of these words, dispute it. Many of the univerals that guide people's thinking and behavior are worth disputing. They simply don't hold up under scrutiny. The three statements listed above are obvious examples. It's possible that caring for Elsie will make it harder to do some of the things she and Michael used to enjoy. But does Alzheimer's make it impossible to ever walk on the beach? They can still go for walks on the beach, only shorter ones. Elsie may need to hold on to Michael's arm, "But the physical contact may feel good and may be good for Elsie, too." In addition, it's obviously not true that all doctors are alike. It's quite possible that Pearl will find one who deals regularly with chronic illness and understand its effects. It's very possible to find a doctor who is accessible and who listens. And when doctors don't respond, there are the nurses to answer questions.

Restrictive statements contain the words *should, have to* and *can't. Should* points to obligations. Some caregivers live with an abundance of *shoulds:* "I should be more patient." "I should be more skilled at caregiving." "I should be able to make better use of my time." "I should be sick, not Dan," says Mark to himself again and again.

The trouble with such statements is that nobody really likes to be "should upon." *Should* statements create a heavy feeling of obligation, one that's enough to wound any relationship. They can be especially hard if they infect the caregiver's relationship with the PWCI. *Should* makes it harder to see choices. People who use a lot of *shoulds* can fall into the trap of feeling they have no choice, that they are victims of forces beyond their control.

Another restrictive phrase is *I can't*. Often a sense of *can't* comes from a core belief system that tells people there is something wrong with them! They believe, in their core, that they are inadequate, incompetent. They feel this way. They feel like they are not okay, like they are incompetent, like they are inadequate.

The key in tackling these limiting thoughts is to try new things and not expect perfection. "Progress not perfection" is a reasonable expectation. There are other creative ways to work limiting words and phrases, as the following applications demonstrate.

Application 55: Taking Action

One simple way to get past *should* is to change the word whenever you use it to *could*. For example, change "I *should* manage my time better" to "I *could* manage my time better." This takes your thinking into a new area. It opens up possibilities, choices, options.

To gain the most benefit from this exercise, follow it up with action. For each *could*, ask how? Take, for example, the statement, "I *should* manage my time better." Follow that up with the question: "How *could* I manage my time better?" Some possible responses: delegate certain tasks to others, dictate memos rather than write them, set a clear stopping time for each meeting. Take action and you will find that you start to shed the victim role.

Application 56: Taking Action

The phrase *have to* presents a case similar to *should,* and the strategy for dealing with it is similar. Substitute the phrase *want to* for *have to* and see where it leads. For example, instead of saying "I *have to* write in my journal each day," try "I *want to* write in my journal each day." Or "I *have to* go to the doctor with Mama" can become "I *want to* go and be there to support her; I know I'll feel better after the visit." Then ask if the new statement rings true for you. If it does, then take action to bring your wants into reality.

Finally, there's the phrase *I can't*. In truth, there are very few things a person can't do. Deep in your heart you feel you can't do a lot of things. That is what you tell yourself. That's what you told yourself for many years. It is hard to break the habit of saying and believing *I can't*.

More often rather than "I can't," what's really going on is "I won't" or "I don't want to" and "I feel like I can't." You truly believe at that time that you can't. Try substituting these phrases for "I can't" and notice how that makes you feel.

Application 57: Taking Action

The key to change, in this case, is to want it. If you really want to change, to do something different, then do it. Even if you feel like you can't. Try it even though it may be difficult. Attempt it even though it may *feel* impossible.

This is crucially important, and it may not come easy. Give it some time.

At times it might seem that habits of negative thinking are "hard-wired" into your brain. These habits are so deeply ingrained that only a kind of artificial shock will disrupt them. One useful way to dispute those thoughts is to take an action that interrupts the pattern, even if it seems a little bizarre. When you detect a wave of negative thinking starting to gain hold in your mind, you could say out loud, "There's that thought" or "Here we go again" or even "Don't listen to that, it'll just make you unhappy." You could even let out a howl, make a face or do a dance step when you feel a wave of negative thinking approaching. Do something harmless — anything — that short-circuits the cycle of negative thinking.

Application 58: Reflecting

Write down three negative thoughts that have occurred to you frequently in the past few weeks. Choose ineffective thoughts — those that deflate your enthusiasm or decrease your options in life. Remember the earlier examples of ineffective thinking: "It's my fault." "This situation won't change." "Things never go well for me."

List your three thoughts.

Now turn those three thoughts around. Rewrite them as ideas that could empower you. Remember the three examples of effective thinking named earlier: "I am not to blame." "I can do something to change this situation — or my attitude toward it." "Even when things go wrong sometimes, my life can go well overall."

List your three new ideas on index cards or stickers.

Now post these thoughts in a place where you'll see them frequently. Repeat them many times each day. Eventually they will become a mental habit — you may even begin to believe them!

Application 59: Taking Action

Choose one "pattern interrupt" you will use to disrupt your negative thoughts. Use it for one week. Has using this technique changed the quality of your thinking? How?

Application 60: Reflecting

Make a list of events in your life that you can control. On a separate page list the events that you truly cannot control. For each item in your can't control list ask, "What prevents me from controlling this?" Then ask if there's anything you can do to overcome that obstacle. Here's how Stella used this exercise.

STELLA, LOLA AND CHRISTINE

Had Stella been raised 30 blocks north and in a different household with different parents, she no doubt would have aspired to a life of the mind, intensity, espresso, sweaters from Bendels in eleven colors, existential crisis. Unfortunately she was raised and lived in the east '40s and intellectually, morally and emotionally she was outfitted by soap operas, TV commercials and *Reader's Digest*.

She sat in her kitchen which had long surrendered both paint and pride and she watched Lola teach Christine the capitalist ethic as they were locked in mortal combat over the Monopoly board. Everywhere in the kitchen, on every surface, were salt and pepper shakers in the shapes of kittens, outhouses, antique telephones, American presidents, shoes, bells, worms, flowers, fruit, religious shrines, the Empire State Building, the Statue of Liberty, the Liberty Bell and the St. Louis Gateway Arches. My God! She enjoyed her collection and decided to go to Second Avenue junk stores to find some new additions.

Stella reflected and verbalized to Lola how stagnant she felt. Lola suggested that while she and Christine engaged in high finance and real estate brokering, Stella might want to make a list of situations in her life that are within her control to change as opposed to things which are not in her control. Stella was motivated. She made a list:

Things that I can't control: Ted's alcoholism, Christine's paralysis, Irene's diabetes, the weather.

Things that are within my control: my boredom and stagnation, this dirty apartment, my response to Ted's drinking.

She and Lola reviewed the list, Lola having been soundly trounced by Christine who had just built hotels on Boardwalk and Park Place. The women decided that they would clean and paint the kitchen which always smelled of cooked cabbage and gas. Cleaning would cost them nothing. She would ask the building superintendent to pay for the paint. Lola would sew new curtains. Maybe Ted could be talked into building shelves to showcase her salt and pepper collection.

"Ted used to love to work with wood. It would involve him in a project and give him something to do besides drink beer and watch TV," said Stella. "And it would certainly eliminate the cluttered look of this room," Lola added. "And I can help wash all the plastic shakers so even if I drop one, it won't break," enthused Christine. "And you can tell Daddy where to put the shakers on the new shelves," Stella added.

"Maybe I can talk Ted into buying one of those ceiling fans on sale at the furniture outlet. They're only $39.00." Stella, Christine and Lola were excited. "I can't control his drinking, but maybe we can do something as a family — have a project with a goal — something that will give us all a sense of accomplishment and not cost a lot of money. And the shiny, clean kitchen will brighten my feelings. We spend so much time in this kitchen," said Stella.

Application 61: Reflecting

The next time you find yourself saying, "I can't do this," ask yourself instead, "What if I could do this?" Follow that with another question: "What prevents me from doing that right now?"

There's a lot to be gained from the "power of positive thinking." In fact, positive thoughts can be especially effective when you let them sink into the depths of your mind and body.

You don't have to express positive thoughts in words. Many times a picture can be just as effective.

To experience this use any relaxation technique that works for you. At the minimum find a quiet, comfortable and private place and close your eyes. Take a deep breath to begin and slowly become aware of your breath. Then just let your body find its own breathing rhythm. Let go of the desire to control your breathing in any way. Let your arms and legs feel light, as if they're floating.

Next, picture a time you spent with your loved one — a happy time, a carefree time when you were together. Now relive that moment in detail. Create the scene using as many sense channels as you can: Remember what you saw, heard, touched, tasted or smelled. Make the mental picture bright, large and vivid in your mind, as if you're adjusting the controls on a wide-screen television set. Then let the scene play itself out and come to its own conclusion. Your only job is to watch it and savor it.

Mark, for example, remembers a Friday night in winter when he and Dan stayed at home simply sitting in front of the fireplace. They didn't say much because there was little need for conversation. "We've spent so much time together that we're connected on a level beyond words," said Mark. "I know that sounds a little flaky, but we both felt it that night. It was one of the few times in my life when I felt no obligation to make conversation. It's great to be that close to someone, to really know someone that well."

Application 62: Working With Feelings

Think about the first time you remember saying, "I can't." What did you feel at that time? Frightened, angry, frustrated or embarrassed?

If you don't remember, move your body in an *I can't* position. For example, stamp your feet, shake your head, squeeze your eyes shut, put your hands over your head. Where do you feel it? In your gut, chest, neck, head, shoulders? What tape plays in your head?

When you care for someone who says, "I can't," what do you react to? How does your body react? Where do you feel it? In your gut, chest, neck, head, shoulders? What tape plays in your head?

Application 63: Taking Action

Find a signal or watchword or symbol indicating *I can't.* Use something nonverbal that you can use to say the words without saying them.

Some words trigger internal responses related to old experiences. By using a signal instead of a word you can let the other person know that for now you don't want to, but eventually you will. Then talk about what's happening.

Pick nonverbal symbols that you can use with your PWCI. For example, tying a purple ribbon on the neck of the dog might symbolize angry feelings. Leaving a cupboard door open might indicate that you're feeling hopeless and downhearted. Closing the cupboard or initiating a conversation would indicate that the intensity of the feelings has subsided.

List some *I can't* situations that come up with your PWCI. For each, list some nonverbal symbols that will work in your household. Remember to share them with your PWCI.

DISTRACT YOURSELF
FROM NEGATIVE THOUGHTS

Positive denial means that no one has to live with the awfulness of chronic illness or caregiving 24 hours each day, seven days each week. Indeed, doing this could wear you out so thoroughly that you'd have little energy left for the person you care for. Working too hard at caregiving can make you an ineffective caregiver.

On any given day, at any moment, you can do whatever is within your ability in order to care for the PWCI. Beyond that you have no obligation to care, nor any further power over chronic illness. No one can reasonably ask you to do more.

The questions to ask become: Who are you when you're not a caregiver? What do you do in your "time off"? Do you define yourself only as a caregiver or as a husband, wife, child, friend?

It's appropriate to engage in healthy distractions. Such distractions are activities other than caregiving that refresh and renew you. It's all right, in fact it's essential, for you to have roles and identities other than caregiver.

There's a sound psychological reason for distraction. It prevents something that therapists call rumination. That word derives from ruminate, meaning "chew the cud," like a cow does when eating. People also ruminate or chew over thoughts in their minds. They can give negative thoughts power over themselves simply by repeating them over and over again or replaying the old tapes. When people dwell on negative thoughts, nurse grudges and harbor resentments, they're doing the emotional equivalent of chewing the cud.

Engaging in healthy distraction is a positive and powerful way to break that habit. When you feel gripped by negative thoughts, try watching TV, reading, jogging, walking, sleeping or doing other activities to escape. When you are distracted from the job of caregiving, allow yourself to stay away mentally and physically for a while. As long as those activities don't lead to undesirable consequences in your life, they can ultimately help you return to the caregiving role with vigor and a fresh perspective.

Application 64: Reflecting

Practice placing different interpretations on events that happen to you. Right now begin with a hypothetical event. If the doctor tells the PWCI that it's time for him or her to start using a wheelchair, can you interpret this event positively? For example: "We've been expecting this for so long, it's actually a relief." "Now I won't have to do so much lifting. Going to a movie will be much easier." Try this with other hypothetical events and with events you're experiencing right now as a caregiver.

Application 65: Reflecting

Experiment with "radical complaining" as a way to dispute negative thoughts. Exaggerate the negative thought until it becomes ridiculous. Say that you're feeling financial stress because of medical bills. Start complaining about money. Talk about how you'll never again be able to afford the things you enjoy. Talk about how you'll be penniless and miserable. Assert that you'll end up out on the street as a homeless person. Keep taking this thought farther and farther until you reach the point of absurdity.

Now, ask if the original negative thought has as much power over you. If so, what is it about that thought that is real? For example, my finances are so tight I can't afford a new car.

CHOOSE YOUR BEHAVIOR

I'd love to change my life totally. Just don't ask me to change any of my habits.

Anonymous

Most of this chapter has concentrated on changing thinking. Changing your thoughts can help you change your feelings and behavior. It's also true that behaving in new ways can help you change your thinking and feeling.

Earlier this book mentioned that you can ask one question of any thought: Is this idea serving me? You can ask similiar questions of any behavior in your life: Is this action serving me? Is it helping me get what I want? Does it increase my effectiveness as a caregiver in the long term?

In changing a behavior, there are three steps that are analogous to steps in changing thinking:

- Detect the old behavior. Just as you notice negative thoughts, notice negative behaviors. To make this observation effective be specific. For example, suppose your goal is to exercise after you eat lunch. If you fail to meet this goal, note precisely what you do instead of exercise: eat a second helping of dessert, nap, read the newspaper, watch TV. Be sure not to judge yourself for failure. Simply observe your behavior in a neutral way, much as a scientist would.
- Dispute the old behavior. That is, pick a new behavior and practice it in place of the old behavior. Be specific. Again, say that you want to get in the habit of exercising after lunch. What exactly will you do: Walk? Jog? Ride a bike? Where will you exercise? Do you need any special equipment or clothing to do this exercise? How will you fit this into your day?
- Distract yourself from the old behavior. Do something else instead — even if it's not the new behavior you want to practice. For instance, instead of taking a nap after lunch, read the paper, go for a walk or take a shower. These actions can help break the old habit, even if you fail to practice the new habit.

One final word: Remember that choosing new thoughts or behaviors does not have to take a long time. Some people are ready for change especially if they are unhappy. Often people are merely waiting for the right idea before they make the leap to a new behavior.

For example, Brenda was able to lose 12 pounds by giving up her habit of eating two desserts every day. Basically she only needed to remember one message whenever she felt the urge to eat sweets: "If you do what you've always done,

you'll receive what you've always received." To her this saying meant: If you eat this dessert again, you'll get the same
old results — extra flab. This saying was so personally vivid
and meaningful that it instantly relieved her of the desire
for those needless calories. The result was a new behavior.
Now she just had to sustain that behavior through another
100 pounds.

Caregiving for a person with chronic illness may force
many changes on you — changes in your thinking as well
as your behavior. Use the ideas and suggestions in this
chapter to avoid being at the mercy of circumstances. Use
them to choose the kind of changes that will keep you sane
as a caregiver.

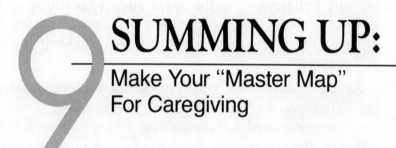

9 SUMMING UP:

Make Your "Master Map" For Caregiving

The Sioux Indians have a saying, "This would be a beautiful, sunny day to die." The person you care for is more than a condition, more than a diagnosis. The person with Alzheimers is a person first — not a problem to solve, not a predicament to fix. Perhaps, in the end, caregiving means only being present, listening, giving attention, loving and remaining open. And in that state of mind the answers will come to you in each moment, as you need them.

CAREGIVERS WANT ANSWERS

Caregivers want to know the right thing to do, the right thing to say when the person they care for is in need. They compare themselves to perfection and they never measure up. They seek a cure and miss opportunities to be helpful.

In reality, the most precious thing you can offer the person with chronic illness, even more than what you do, is who you are. Ultimately what you give is not medication, relief or distraction — it's moment-by-moment attention. It's vision and values. You can't fix, but you can listen. You can't cure, but you can care. You can simply stay present to whatever happens — knowing it precisely, accepting it fully. You can be with chronic illness.

Putting this into practice is not easy. Being with chronic illness means putting yourself into a certain state of mind. In that state effective words and actions flow naturally, doing flows from being. It means becoming a "human being" not a "human doing."

Approach caregiving with a mind that is alert and accepting. When you do, you start to let go gently of the negative emotions associated with caregiving. These emotions — pity, self-pity, the compulsive need to "fix" or cure the person with chronic illness, co-dependent behaviors — are the ripples on the lake. They are the dirt that clouds the mirror. When you go into the observer state, you calm the torrent of worry, fear and pity. You clean the mirror. And when the mirror is clean, you can see more clearly what is — not what should be. Seeing that, you can choose your actions. What you're doing is staying in the present moment. There will be many times when your attention will wander, when you fantasize about the future or rue the past and you don't have to beat yourself up about it. You just need to practice coming back to the present.

Steven Levine is a person trained in meditation and known for his work with dying people. He calls the process he works with "conscious dying." The first step in that process, he says, is seeing that people are not their bodies. But, even more, it's seeing how your experience changes in every second. "To let go of the last moment and open to the next is to die consciously," writes Levine.

It's this kind of death — not death of the physical body — that comes into play when you stay present to the process. When you let go of your answers, your desire for things to stay the same, then you're letting go of the last moment. And as you open to the next one, the answers will come to you as you need them.

MAKING A SKILLBOX

This book suggests techniques and explains many skills, especially in the applications sprinkled throughout. And all of them have a single goal: Helping you take care of yourself as you care for a person with a chronic illness.

Don't become too attached to gaining skills. Some caregivers may seek to apply the suggestions provided with a kind of perfectionism that defeats the purpose of this book. That plunges them farther into worry when they fail to measure up to their own rising expectations. They get into trouble if they hold on to specific expectations, rather than acquiring skills which are general and flexible.

Instead, use a toolbox — or more appropriately — a "skillbox." Put in your skillbox a repertoire of tips and techniques for lifting your spirits and inciting constructive action. Sometimes, however, boxes can get so stuffed with ideas that you start to feel overloaded. When you try to keep track of so many options, you run the danger of losing your spontaneity and seasoned judgment. You start playing by the rule book and forget about your primary goal which is to be a good caregiver.

Developing certain skills can help you feel better and increase your effectiveness as a caregiver. Yet a tool or technique that works well in one situation or with one person can fail in a different situation or with a different person. In order to stay sane you need to learn which skill to use at a given time. How do you choose?

Many things come into play in making this decision, including your past experience, your knowledge, your hunches and your guesses. But mostly, it is your moment-by-moment attention. By staying present to what is going on right now, both for yourself and the PWCI, you are staying present to the process. It's probably the most valuable tool a caregiver can have.

Healthy caregiving involves finding balance. It's choosing a path between extremes. Actually, there is probably a time for all the suggestions in this book — and for their opposites. Sometimes people implore, question, argue, challenge, cry or scream. At other times people are quiet, forgiving. Staying present to the process means observing each emotion, experiencing it and responding to it at the time it occurs.

What is the PWCI feeling and thinking right now? What is the one thing I feel most strongly? What does my "gut" tell me is the right thing to do at this moment? What can I do that would really help? When you're too busy chasing answers, you can keep such questions from surfacing. Unless you pay attention to the questions, you have little hope of finding answers. Letting the questions come to the surface promotes healing. It pushes caregiving to a new level of effectiveness — even when you don't know the answers.

THE MASTER MAP

Another way to help take care of yourself is to make a "master map" of your ideas and intentions related to caregiving. This will help you get a clear picture of the main ideas you've picked up from this book, and it will represent those ideas in a way that you'll remember and be able to use.

This can be fun and a great way to integrate new ideas into your mind and heart. You can make lists, draw pictures — anything that represents this material in a vivid way for you.

Keep in mind the purpose of a map. A map helps you find your way when you're lost or when you're encountering territory for the first time. Caregiving might leave you feeling lost, and it can take you to many new places in your life. If that happens, a map of key ideas and suggestions can help you get your bearings. If you've been somewhere before, it helps you retrace your steps accurately. It enables you to choose alternative routes you might take.

One example of a master map comes from Evy McDonald, a nurse who was diagnosed with a terminal illness in 1980 and given one year to live. She used this time to examine and reorient her life. The transformation that took place in her led to the disappearance of her disease. McDonald sums up her experience with:

SEVEN KEYS TO TRUE HEALING

1. **From get to give: demanding from life to giving to life.** Preoccupation with what one can get — even getting well! — keeps one stuck in a small world, separated from others and thus from the experience of love. When the emphasis shifts to giving, the self opens up to a more spacious arena of connectedness with others and a greater feeling of aliveness that endures no matter what the physical outcome of the disease. True service heals the server.

2. **From expecting and preparing for death to celebrating life and living every moment.** Life is to be lived. Whether circumstances are radiant health or a terminal illness, people are all mortal and could die tomorrow. It is the quality of life that is important, not the quantity. A life fully lived, moment-to-moment, is health-enhancing on all levels. A preoccupation with death, be it physical death or the day-in, day-out petty type of existence, can only detract from overall well-being.

3. **From resentment to forgiveness: forgiving self and others.** Resentment is poison. Taking offense and holding in the anger and frustration often erupts in mental

or physical disease. Forgiveness is the act of changing the perception of the offense, of taking a larger, less personal view of the situation; it re-establishes harmony and preserves health.

4. **From self-pity and self-hatred to self-acceptance and unconditional self-love.** When a person hates his or her body — the big hips, bald head, flabby arms, ugly nose — the body, the mirror of thoughts, may respond by becoming ill. Not to accept any aspect of life (including what a person doesn't like about his or her body) is to deny life. To accept and love one's body is to affirm life.

5. **From wanting to escape from life to accepting life exactly as it is.** Children often use the excuse of a stomache ache to avoid going to school. That is not too different from the woman who develops cancer because she is too afraid to leave the marriage she hates. Or the heart attack "victim" who, for years, has felt trapped in an unsatisfying job and wanted out. Leaving "dead-end" circumstances consciously, through realistic assessment and compassionate means, is life-affirming and life-enhancing. Accepting life just as it is — including a chronic illness — allows life to restore health.

6. **From denial of painful emotions to sharing them and letting them go.** Denying emotions, especially painful or negative ones, is a certain kind of hypocrisy that is difficult to maintain without a good deal of internal stress. When such feelings are unacknowledged, they find expression in devious and unhealthy ways, including physical illness. While a person doesn't need to dramatize these feelings, simply acknowledging them and sharing them dilutes their power and makes it possible to let them go.

7. **From avoidance of intimacy to opening the self to love.** To build a protective barrier around one's self, closing one's self to intimacy, is to affirm one's separateness, isolation and thus deny one's self the life-giving energy

of connectedness to others. Everyone has experienced how good it can feel to open up some protected corner of themselves and be close to another person. That good feeling is an important component of health — love is the ultimate healing power.

Even though McDonald originally formulated these principles from the perspective of someone with an illness, they apply equally to caregivers. Your map does not have to be nearly as long or as sophisticated. A simple list of affirmations, posted on the wall or written individually on index cards, may be enough:

> I take time for myself regularly.
> I choose thoughts that promote my well-being.
> I choose behaviors that promote my well-being.
> I eat food that promotes my health.
> I exercise three times each week.
> I separate the person from that person's hurtful words or actions.

Another form for your map to take is a simple "laundry list" of the key ideas. Remember to include the ideas that will help you most in day-to-day caregiving. For example, the core assertions of this book are:

- Staying present to the process.
- Taking care of yourself helps you be a better caregiver.
- Connecting takes work, and it's worth it.
- Chronic illness is about changing.
- Everything is going to be all right. All is well.

Following are some applications to help you design your personal caregiving road map.

Application 66: Learning

Consider what you've read in this book and look over your responses to the applications. In light of all this, what are the three most important things you can take away from this book?

What ideas or tools will make a difference in your life? Write those ideas in three sentences.

Now, list some specific ways you can apply these ideas to your day-to-day caregiving. Be specific. What will you do differently? How will you know that a change has taken place in your life?

Application 67: Taking Action

List four or five goals you want to attain after using this book. Express them in one sentence each.

Now look over your list. Is there any way to combine these goals, to pursue two or more of them at one time? For example, if your goal is to exercise daily and to see close friends more often, can you choose one friend to exercise with? If your goal is to read more and widen your circle of friends, consider starting a small book discussion group.

Application 68: Taking Action

Make a chart that represents your overall plan for caregiving. Divide a large sheet of paper into three columns. Label the first column "What the PWCI Wants." Label the second column "What I Want." And label the last column "Resources For Getting What We Want." This exercise will be more powerful if you are specific with each item you list. If you want to ask for money, name a specific amount. If you want help from your family, list specific caregiving tasks they can do. Be realistic.

Consider filling out this chart with the PWCI, as well as any friends and family members who will take part in caregiving.

Application 69: Taking Action

Imagine that you ask for and receive any caregiving help you wanted from your close friends and family members. What are three things you would ask for? List those things and who you would ask for each one.

Now look over your list and consider asking for these things, even if they seem outlandish at first.

Application 70: Learning

Make a "map" of the most important ideas you got from this book. Write the word "caregiving" in the center of a blank, unlined piece of paper. Then, on branches radiating out from the center, write single words or short phrases that sum up each important idea. Create further branches expressing related ideas and subtopics. Here's an example:

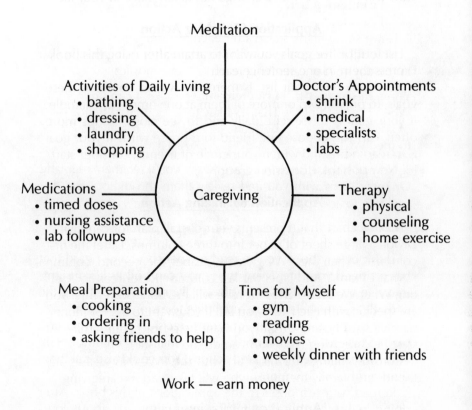

Meditation

Activities of Daily Living
• bathing
• dressing
• laundry
• shopping

Doctor's Appointments
• shrink
• medical
• specialists
• labs

Medications
• timed doses
• nursing assistance
• lab followups

Caregiving

Therapy
• physical
• counseling
• home exercise

Meal Preparation
• cooking
• ordering in
• asking friends to help

Time for Myself
• gym
• reading
• movies
• weekly dinner with friends

Work — earn money

Application 71: Learning

Take a stack of index cards and write three phrases on each card:

When this happens:
I can remember:
I can do:

Leave some blank space after each phrase.

Now, fill in these blanks with some specifics that can help you in the day-to-day caregiving routine. For example:

When this happens:	I can remember:	I can do:
When I can't think of anything to say to the PWCI	That it's okay to be silent	Hold hands — reach out

Now post these cards in a place where you'll see them regularly. Or carry them with you and review them throughout the day. Feel free to add to them at any time.

Application 72: Reflecting

Think of any book you've read or speech you've heard that has changed your life. Many times you can boil its key insights into a few sentences, paragraphs or diagrams. These bring the core ideas into sharp focus, much like focusing a camera.

Part of this is making a conscious decision about what you plan to take away from a book. Often what you remember falls into two categories: ideas and actions. You could also call them discoveries and intentions.

Reread your responses to the applications in this book. After doing so, list the three main discoveries you made about yourself as a caregiver.

Now list the three most important actions you intend to take as a result of reading this book. These are actions you intend to carry out no matter what.

Consider sharing these discoveries and intentions with the person you care for, and ask for that person's support.

ROSE, ELSIE AND MICHAEL

Michael was beside himself. Elsie had wandered out of the apartment while Michael was showering. She had wandered off and had been missing for six hours. Michael, after calling the Miami police and being told he could not file a missing person report for 24 hours, phoned Rose and Paul. This was the last straw. Even Michael had to agree that things were out of control. Rose was on the evening plane and Paul would arrive late the next evening. Michael would locate his beloved Elsie in a police station. She had been missing for 38 hours. Elsie was totally disoriented and did not recognize any members of her family. There was no doubt in anyone's mind that it was time for her to be placed in a nursing home. Michael would go with her. They would get a double room.

"Isn't it funny how things work out?" Rose was saying to her brother. "Seventy-two hours ago it would have been easier to explain quantum radiation in a foreign language than to get Pa to agree to put Ma in a nursing home." As much as he hated to admit it, Paul had to agree with Rose. It had taken a major crisis and the Miami police to get the old man to agree to go into a nursing home with his wife. But he would not give up their condo.

Rose would leave Park Avenue's pitch of urbanity and roar of ritz for one week a month. It was during that week that Michael would bring Elsie back to the condo. Rose, Elsie and Michael would take the long walks along the ocean each morning that meant so much to Elsie and Michael. And they would gather shells to add to their collection. They'd have an early lunch on the balcony and an early bird dinner. Michael would schmooze with his cronies or play cards in the game room of the building while Rose looked after her mother.

When it was time for Rose to return to New York and time for Elsie to be taken back to the nursing home, Michael would offer some resistance, but would always give in because he'd know, down deep, that Elsie had become too much for him to handle alone. Elsie's final wandering episode had been one of many, but Michael had always been able to find her within an hour or two. That last episode knocked some sense into him. Besides, he was able to be with Elsie in the nursing home and because of the close supervision, Michael was able to make some new friends over shuffleboard and canasta. And Elsie loved the daily swimnastics in the pool. She couldn't remember the routines, but she loved the music, the splashing and the laughter.

Paul promised to make more frequent trips to visit his parents in Miami. But somehow Rose was not optimistic about this actually happening. She had come to realize and was resigned to the fact that family trouble was the worst kind and it seemed that she and Paul ran their own version of the Middle East. At least he had agreed to pay half the expenses and her parents were safe, guarded and in good hands.

In Rose's last session of the season with Dr. Wilburforce (he was off to Fire Island for the summer) she shared her inventory of the past six months from her journal. "I'm amazed I've learned so much. I've become painfully aware of my selfishness and I've actually begun to change! I'm less intolerant of Paul's limitations and of my own. I've learned about acceptance, forgiveness and patience. But I still wish the beast (that was how she now referred to Paul's wife . . . better than some of the four-letter words she had used to use) would drop dead."

She read the last part with a smirk, knowing it would get her psychiatrist's attention. "Yes, Rose dear, we can pick up there in September."

STELLA, LOLA AND CHRISTINE

Between the exhortations of Lola and the sympathy of some neighbors, Stella was able to gather enough traction to spin her tires out of the mud. Although interacting as a family and even as husband and wife was as rare as finding pearls in a box of cereal, the clean-up, paint-up, fix-up-the-kitchen project had moved Ted and Stella and even Christine out of the doldrums.

Stella looked around the kitchen. Her stove and refrigerator, once shrines of neglect, were glistening, thanks to Lola and a neighbor. Ted had built shelves and shadow boxes for Stella's shaker collection, alleviating the clutter. The curtains Lola had sewn brightened the place, as did the new bright colored paint. And she got the ceiling fan she wanted, literally and figuratively bringing a breath of fresh air into the room where she, Christine, Irene and Lola spent so much of their time.

Stella had learned over the past few months that, although some things in her life could not be reversed, there were things over which she had control. The small change in her living space brightened her life. She learned that there were still things they could do as a family. All she'd have to do was exercise some creativity, keep her eyes and mind open, suggest and initiate. Ted would not initiate so it was always up to her. She was often surprised that he frequently agreed to do what she'd ask or suggest. Stella also learned that she could have outside interests — in her case weekly bowling and an NA meeting. These limited activities would not compromise the care of her sick children.

Life was tough for Stella and Lola, but they rallied as always. They were survivors. And in the face of chronic illness they had the essential traits of caregivers who survive: Willingness to change and grow in the face of adversity.

DAN AND MARK

Dan had been in the hospital for three weeks, submitted to every medieval torture. Tomorrow Mark would bring him home. The swollen and dizzy autumn moon — the color of nectarines — shone through the hospital window.

Four days earlier Dan had decided to cultivate a moustache. Wispy little whiskers, as skinny and forlorn as African cattle,

wandered the plain beneath his nose. Mark stared at his
dozing friend and at the whiskers and chuckled. "What's so
amusing?" Dan asked smiling. Mark thought that his lover's
smile was golden and that his voice had not lost a calorie of
its old blue heat. "I was just picturing what you'll look like
with a moustache, and I was thinking how good it will be to
have you back home. Tommy and Jay want to come over
tomorrow night and cook a little something for you."

"A little something? That'll be the day! Those guys have
more words for overeating than Eskimos have for snow and
the Japanese have for no." They both laughed.

Over the next week the phone was constant with Phyllis'
and friends' concern. It was a relief to have Dan's mother out
of the house and back in New Jersey, even though Mark had
come to grips with her intrusiveness and abrasiveness. After
all, she only had what she thought to be her son's best interests at heart. But with her gone the men could talk more
freely. They acknowledged that they subscribed to the old
medical chestnut — hope for the best, prepare for the worst.
And prepare they did. Dan for the first time talked about his
wake and funeral. Always a clotheshorse, he would leave
instructions with the undertaker to change his suits twice a
day so that he was not seen in the same suit twice. Dan and
Mark laughed at the absurdity of the idea, but it would be so
outrageously typical of Dan. "Let's keep them laughing to the
end," laughed Dan. Over the next weeks more serious details
were outlined.

The last stay at the hospital had taken a severe toll. Dan
had crossed a mine field and the price he paid to get through
to the other side was that he'd need to sleep an hour for an
hour of strength. "I'm so sorry I'm putting you through this,
Mark. You mean everything to me and I hate to see how
burdensome I am. I feel that the parade is passing you by and
that I am responsible for you not being in it," said Dan.

Mark told Dan a story about Diogenes. Diogenes' sole
possession was a tin cup from which he drank water from a

well. One day he saw a beggar scooping water with his cupped hands and Diogenes then threw away his cup because he too knew he could drink with his hands. "It turns out there is no end to learning what you can do without," said Mark, assuring Dan that the sacrifices were insignificant compared to the time they had together.

PEARL, RITA AND JACKIE

Rita was sitting in bed watching her mother and daughter prepare for Rita's fourth trip to the hospital during the past few months. The doctor indicated that this might be a very long stay. When they pressed him about "how long" during his afternoon house call, he was almost playful. Both his playfulness and the house call were firsts in Dr. Ratner's cool demeanor. "I always say three to four weeks because my father was a tailor. He used to say, 'You can cut the pants too long, but never cut them too short.' "

Pearl showed the doctor to the elevator. Dr. Ratner told Pearl that he was concerned about Rita's lack of response to the latest round of chemotherapy. And he was even more concerned about how toxic this set of drugs had been to her system. The oozing of blood from her gums was a sign that her platelets had been wiped out. If her white blood cells suffered a similar fate, there was a possibility that she might not make it out of the hospital. He had always been painfully honest and tonight was no exception.

Rita was returning to the famous teaching hospital, the kind that generates income and attracts interesting cases. The caliber of its medical staff had a history of exciting the philanthropic impulses of the rich, who wanted to make sure it was the right place in which to be sick. At least Rita would be well taken care of there. When the doctor left, Joey climbed onto his mother's bed with a book they had been reading together — *Robinson Crusoe*. "What an appropriate book," said Rita. "This is the story of our lives. Surviving a terrible storm at sea; then being shipwrecked; waking from catastrophe and finding ourselves alone in a new, alien world. Even though we are all here, we have our own personal, individual experiences of this adventure. And the past year's experience has strengthened us and toughened us and brought us closer together."

For a moment, Rita reflected on the caregiving styles of Pearl and Jackie: Pearl — endlessly gentle, easing the difficult symptoms, always comforting, making light of every indignity, never letting the fear of heartbreak twist her up; and Jackie, now 17, still ranting and screaming in free falls of rage — a reaction that had become a reflex — at every little thing that went wrong in the world of school, boyfriends, errands and customer service. It was pure displacement and they all realized it. Jackie was still angry at Rita for being sick, but not as angry as she had been.

Rita looked at her mother and daughter. They were confident and calm, and so was she. She wasn't sure whether this calmness was patience or resignation. But impatient Joey interrupted her thoughts. He wanted to get on with *Robinson Crusoe*. Rita and Joey snuggled up to one another as the women finished packing. It was almost time to get on with their personal adventure.

Rita was thankful to Mrs. Goodwell, the school counselor, who had helped her family so much. She admired the dedication of such professionals. Pearl and Jackie talked openly about the anger, resentment, deprivation, pain and fear. This was so comforting to Rita because she knew that even if she wasn't coming back from the hospital this time, Pearl, Jackie and Joey would be all right.

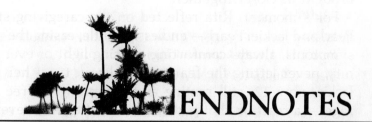

ENDNOTES

Introduction

1. Mayerhoff, Milton. **On Caring.** New York, New York: Harper & Row, 1971, p. 2.

2. Pohl, Mel, Kay, Deniston, Toft, Doug. **The Caregivers' Journey.** Center City, MN: Hazelden, 1990, p. 40-42.

Chapter 1

1. Pohl, Mel, Kay, Deniston, Toft, Doug. **The Caregivers' Journey,** p. 40-42.

Chapter 2

1. Pohl, Mel, Kay, Deniston, Toft, Doug. **The Caregivers' Journey,** p. 116-119.

Chapter 3

1. From Attneave, Carol, Ph.D., c/o Fred Duhl, Boston Family Institute, 251 Harvard St., Brookline, MA 02146.

2. Smith, Huston. **Religions of Man.** New York: Harper & Row, 1958, p. 88.

3. Cousins, Norman. **Anatomy of an Illness.** New York: Norton, 1979, p. 71-73.

4. Fisher, Roger. **Getting To Yes.** Boston: Houghton-Mifflin, 1991, p. 15.

5. Seigel, Bernie, M.D. **Love, Medicine and Miracles.** New York: Harper & Row, 1986, p. 22-26.

Chapter 4

1. Woititz, Janet Geringer. **Adult Children of Alcoholics.** Pompano Beach, FL: Health Communications, 1983, p. 4-5.

2. Black, Claudia. **It Will Never Happen To Me!** Denver: M.A.C., 1982, p. 31.

3. A., Tony with Dan F. **The Laundry List: The ACoA Experience.** Deerfield Beach, FL: Health Communications, 1991, p. viii.

4. Williamson, Marian. **Return To Love: Reflections on the Principles of A Course in Miracles.** New York: Harper Collins, 1992, p. 28.

5. Levine, Stephen. **Who Dies?** Garden City, NY: Doubleday/Anchor Press, 1982, p. 52.

6. Roger, John & McWilliams, Peter. **You Can't Afford The Luxury Of A Negative Thought.** Los Angeles: Prelude Press, 1990, p. 54.

7. Boerstler, Richard. **Letting Go: A Holistic and Meditative Approach to Living and Dying.** South Yarmouth, MA: Associates of Thanatology Press, 1982, p. 27-40.

Chapter 5

1. Pennebaker, James. "Writing Your Wrongs". *American Health,* January/February 1991, p. 64-67.

2. Garfield, Patricia. "The Healing Power Of Dreams". *New Age Journal,* June 1991, p. 36.

Chapter 6

1. Easwaran, Eknath. **Meditation: An Eight Point Program.** Petaluma, California: Nilgiri, 1978, p. 23.

Chapter 7

1. Kalidasa, from **The Slogans: Basic Tools for Recovery.** Center City, MN: Hazelden, 1990, p. 23.

Chapter 8

1. Frankl, Viktor. **Man's Search For Meaning.** New York: Simon & Schuster, 1984, p. 86.

2. Pohl, Mel, Kay, Deniston, Toft, Doug. **The Caregivers' Journey.** Center City, MN: Hazelden, 1990, p. 206-207.

Chapter 9

1. From McDonald, Evy, New Road Map Foundation, Seattle: 1990.

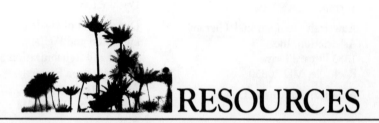

RESOURCES

Adult Day Care Associations
(consult your local directory or
call your local United Way)

**Alcoholics Anonymous Control
World Service**
P.O. Box 459
Grand Central Station, NY 10163

Alzheimer's Association
70 East Lake Street
Suite 600
Chicago, IL 60601

**American Association of Marriage
and Family Counselors**
225 Yale Avenue
Claremont, CA 91711

**American Association on
Mental Deficiency**
1719 Kalorama Road, N.W.
Washington, D.C. 20009

American Cancer Society
777 Third Avenue
New York, NY 10017

**American Coalition of
Citizens with Disabilities**
1200 15th Street, N.W.
Suite 201
Washington, D.C. 20005

**American Diabetes Association
National Service Center**
1160 Duke Street
P.O. Box 25757
Alexandria, VA 22314

American Geriatric Society
10 Columbus Circle
Suite 1470
New York, NY 10019

**American Heart Association
National Office**
7320 Greenville Avenue
Dallas, TX 75231

American Lung Association
1740 Broadway
New York, NY 10019

American Lupus Society,
National Office
23751 Madison Street
Torrance, CA 90505

American Occupational Therapy
Association, Inc.
1383 Piccard Drive
Rockville, MD 20850

American Parkinson Disease
Association
116 John Street
New York, NY 10038

American Physical Therapy
Association
1156 15th Street, N.W.
Washington, D.C. 20009

American Psychological Association
1200 17th Street, N.W.
Washington, D.C. 20036

The Amyotrophic Lateral
Sclerosis Association
185 Madison Avenue, Suite 1001
P.O. Box 2130
New York, NY 10016

Arthritis Foundation
National Office
1314 Spring Street, N.W.
Atlanta, GA 30309

The Association for the
Severely Handicapped
7010 Roosevelt Way, N.E.
Seattle, WA 98115

Asthma Care Association
of America
P.O. Box 568
Spring Valley Road
Ossining, NY 10562

Clearinghouse on the Handicapped
Office of Special Education and
Rehabilitative Services
Department of Education
Room 3106, Switzer Building
330 C Street, S.W.
Washington, D.C. 20202

Department of Health,
Education and Welfare
Social and Rehabilitation Services
Rehabilitation Service
Administration
Washington, D.C. 20014

Epilepsy Foundation of America
4351 Garden Drive
Suite 406
Landover, MD 20785

Gerontogolocial Society
Clinical Medicine Section
1 Dupont Circle
Washington, D.C. 20036

Guillaume-Barre Syndrome
Support Group
P.O. Box 262
Wynnewood, PA 19096

Hospice Organizations
(consult your local directory or
call your local United Way)

Library of Congress
Division for the Blind and
Physically Handicapped
Washington, D.C. 20542

Muscular Dystrophy Association,
National Office
810 Seventh Avenue
New York, NY 10019

Myasthenia Gravis Foundation, Inc.
7-11 South Broadway, Suite 304
White Plains, NY 10601

**National Association of
People with AIDS**
2025 I Street, N.W.
Suite 1118
Washington, D.C. 20006

**National Association of the
Physically Handicapped**
2810 Terrace Road, S.E.
Washington, D.C. 20020

National Cancer Institute
9000 Rockville Pike
Bethesda, MD 20892
For info: call 1-800-4-CANCER
For pamphlets: 1-800-638-6694

National Council on Alcoholism
12 West 21st
New York, NY 10010

**National Lesbian & Gay
Health Foundation**
P.O. Box 65472
Washington, D.C. 20035

**National Lupus Erythematosus
Foundation**
5430 Van Nuys Boulevard
Suite 206
Van Nuys, CA 91401

**National Multiple Sclerosis
Society, National Office**
733 3rd Avenue, 6th Floor
New York, NY 10017

**National Organization for
Rare Disorders, Inc.**
P.O. Box 8923
New Fairfield, CT 06812

**National Self-Help Clearinghouse
Graduate School & University Cntr.
of the City University of New York**
33 West 42nd Street
Room 1227
New York, NY 10036

**Parkinson's Educational Program
(PEP*USA)**
1800 Park Newport, #302
Newport Beach, CA 92660
*(A wide variety of products and informa-
tion resources; write for complete catalog
and newsletter)*

**Sex Information and Education
Council of the U.S. (SIECUS)
New York University Resource
Center and Library**
51 West 4th Street
New York, NY 10003
*(This is an excellent resource for lay people
and professionals. Request the complete list
of available topics.)*

Tourette Syndrome Association
41-02 Bell Boulevard
Bayside, NY 11361

Organizations And National Offices, Canada

**ALS Society of Canada
(Amyotrophic Lateral Sclerosis)**
250 Rogers Road
Toronto, Ontario MGE 1R1
Canada

Arthritis Society (Canada)
920 Yonge Street
Suite 420
Toronto, Ontario, M4W 3J7
Canada

**Canadian National Institute
for the Blind**
1931 Bayview Avenue
Toronto, Ontario M4G 4C8
Canada

Canadian Association for the Deaf
2395 Bayview Avenue
Willowdale, Ontario M2L 1A2
Canada

Canadian Cancer Society
130 Bloor Street West
Suite 1001
Toronto, Ontario M5S 2V7
Canada

**Canadian Cystic Fibrosis
Foundation**
586 Eglinton Avenue East
Suite 204
Toronto, Ontario M5S 1N5
Canada

Canadian Diabetes Association
78 Bond Street
Toronto, Ontario M5B 2J8
Canada

**Canadian Heart and Stroke
Foundation**
1 Nicholas Street
Suite 1200
Ottawa, Ontario K1N 7B7
Canada

Canadian Lung Association
75 Albert Street
Suite 908
Ottawa, Ontario K1P 5E7
Canada

Epilepsy Ontario
2160 Yonge Street, First Floor
Toronto, Ontario M4S 2A9
Canada

**Lupus Foundation of
Ontario Corporation**
P.O. Box 687
289 Ridge Road North
Ridgeway, Ontario L0S 1N0
Canada

Multiple Sclerosis Society of Canada
130 Bloor Street West
Suite 700
Toronto, Ontario M5S 1S5
Canada

**Muscular Dystrophy Association
of Canada**
367 Bay Street, Tenth Floor
Toronto, Ontario M5H 2T7
Canada

**Ontario March of Dimes
(Crippling Illnesses)**
60 Overlea Boulevard
Toronto, Ontario M5H 2T7
Canada

**National AIDS Committee Ministry
of National Health & Welfare**
Ottawa, Ontario K1A 0K9
Canada

Parkinson Foundation of Canada
232 Bloor Street West
Toronto, Ontario M4W 1A6
Canada